Vegan Diet For Athletes

A plant-based nutrition guide for vegan

Understanding vegan diet

Thomas Felling

Table of Contents

Prologue

"My job is to be fit and I am really blessed that I get to go and work out and live a healthy lifestyle."

The words of Kerri Walsh, an American professional beach volleyball player, shows how important following a healthy and balanced diet is, especially in the world of sports. It is a fact that athletes need to sustain energy levels that exceed the ones an average person needs for his or her everyday activities. For this reason, athletes need to follow a balanced diet that provides their bodies with all the nutrients they need and thus allowing them to perform their best at their respective sport. Up until now, it was a widely held belief that animal products were the best source for people to acquire the necessary nutrients for their diet and thus, meat was a "must" on any dietary plan, especially in the sports world.

However, many athletes have decided to follow a different path, a path that shows animal products are not a necessity for them to get the much-needed nutrients to perform their best. This shift, which is the main subject of this book, has to do with the growing number of athletes following a vegan diet and eliminating animal products from their dietary schedule while still getting all the optimal nutrients (such as proteins, carbohydrates and fats) they need to stay in shape and perform their best at the sport of their choice.

Actually, the belief and practice of veganism has existed for many years and has been practiced consistently by many people all over the world. There are many reports of both men and women who have eliminated animal products from their lives and have successfully stayed healthy by getting all the nutrients their body needs. In this book, we will analyze how the vegan diet applies to the world of sports and present some of the most famous athletes that have decided to indulge in this lifestyle.

In the first chapter, we will provide you with the necessary information to get a better grasp of what a diet is and of how a balanced and healthy diet can benefit an average person. For this chapter only, we will mention a complete guide including meat products. The rest of the book will focus solely on the vegan diet. In the second chapter, we will analyze the different levels of vegetarianism as well as the different food groups to provide you with a better understanding on the meaning and practice of vegetarianism and its subcategories. In the third chapter we will present you with the various reasons people, and especially athletes, choose to make an important turn in their lives and adopt a vegan lifestyle as well as provide you with an overall analysis on the vegan philosophy. In the fourth chapter, we will offer some information and guidelines that will help you make the transition from an omnivorous diet to a vegan one easier. There are many cases of people who tried to adopt a vegan diet and lifestyle but failed because they rushed this transition or have done so with the thought of simply losing weight; veganism is much more than just a diet.

In the fifth chapter, we will analyze the various ways athletes could obtain all the nutrients they need while following a vegan diet and present one of the most known athletes that became vegan and encouraged, as well as inspired, many people to do so: Lewis Hamilton. There are many people, particularly sports coaches that doubt the fact that a vegan diet could provide the necessary nutrients for an athlete to achieve their optimal health and performance. This is the myth we will try to deal with in this chapter and present the basic guidelines through which athletes could follow a vegan diet safely and without worrying about diminishing their health and performance.

In the sixth chapter, we are going to present you with the various sources you will be able to get the necessary nutrition and offer some general guidelines on sports nutrition for athletes to be able to train better with the provided nutrients. In the seventh and final chapter, we will give the athletes some advice on sports nutrition, provide them with a sample meal plan for a day and suggest a few recipes that are included in the sample meal plan. Let us begin our journey!

Understanding the Word "Diet"

Believe it or not, each person follows a diet. Each person has a pattern or a way he or she eats almost every day. For example, you may follow a diet that is full of fried chicken, donuts and sugary drinks or you may follow a diet that contains cheese, pasta and meat or even a diet based on nonfat dairy products, fresh salads and grilled fish. Those three diets will offer you nutrients such as fats, carbohydrates and proteins, but each diet plan will have a different effect on your body. What differentiates a balanced and healthy way of eating from a bad and unbalanced one is consuming, on a daily basis, a wide variety of nutritious foods and, at the same time, keeping an appropriate level of calories for your body. To better understand how this concept works, let us start with the basics.

Every food we consume has nutrients. These are defined as molecules, or else compounds, found in food that each organism on this planet needs to develop, produce energy, reproduce, repair and grow. When we digest nutrients, they are broken down by the organism into different parts that are later used by it. Keep in mind that the human body is not able to create nutrients on its own and, for this reason, it should acquire those from the diet each person follows. This makes our eating habits essential since a poor intake of nutrients will result in poor health. In the food we will also find non-nutrients that have the potential to harm our bodies such as preservatives, cholesterol and dyes, as well as helpful non-nutrients such as antioxidants and omega-3 fatty acids

Nutrients are separated into six classes that include:

- ✓ Lipids

- ✓ Water

- ✓ Carbohydrates

- ✓ Proteins

- ✓ Minerals

- ✓ Vitamins

Those six classes can be further categorized into two groups, the Macronutrients and Micronutrients. Macronutrients include the nutrients that we need in abundance and they are:

- ✓ Proteins

- ✓ Carbohydrates

- ✓ Lipids

- ✓ Water

The above can be processed by our metabolism into cellular energy and this energy stems from the chemical bonds of those nutrients. When this chemical energy is metabolized into cellular energy, we can perform our basic functions. The energy that is found in our food can be measured with calories. When we read the nutrition labels of various foods, the number that corresponds to calories is produced by multiplying by one thousand each calorie. Also, water is considered a macronutrient because we need to take in large amounts of it on a daily basis, but it has no calories unlike the rest of the macronutrients.

Proteins are large molecules built from chains of amino acids which in turn are defined as the building blocks of proteins. Amino acids are created from nitrogen, oxygen, hydrogen, and carbon and more than 20 different combinations of amino acids can be used to build proteins we can find in nature. There are two basic classes of amino acids: we have the non-essential amino acids, which the human body is able to produce, and then we have the essential amino acids. The latter need to be introduced in the human body which is not able to produce them on its own.

Our bodies require proteins for the function, regulation and structure of the cells as well as the proper function of organs and tissues. They are also essential for the structure of muscles, bones, and skin as well as carrying out a lot of the chemical reactions that happen in the human body. Proteins offer 4 kilocalories of energy per gram and are found in abundance in animal products such as seafood, dairy products and meat or in plant foods such as nuts, soy and beans.

The amount of proteins a person needs usually depends on their health, weight and age. In general, the recommended dietary intake when it comes to proteins is:

- ✓ 46 grams for adult women
- ✓ 56 grams for adult men

- ✓ Approximately 1 g/kg for women who are pregnant or breastfeeding, as well as for women and men who are over 70 years of age.

According to experts, there are over one hundred thousand different proteins that reside in our bodies. Generally, the main sources of proteins are dairy products, fish, tofu, eggs and meat. The following foods are rich in proteins and are found in many balanced dietary plans :

- ✓ Eggs: 6 grams of proteins in one large egg and 78 calories

- ✓ Almonds: 6 grams of proteins per 28g and 161 calories

- ✓ Chicken Breast: 53 grams of proteins for 1 chicken breast that is roasted and without skin and it contains 284 calories.

- ✓ Oats: 13 grams of proteins on half a cup of uncooked oats and 303 calories.

- ✓ Cottage Cheese: 27 grams of proteins in 226g of cottage cheese that contains 2% fat and has 194 calories.

- ✓ Greek Yogurt: 17 grams of proteins in 170g and 100 calories in non-fat Greek yogurt.

- ✓ Milk: 8 grams of proteins in a cup of whole milk and 149 calories.

- ✓ Broccoli: 3 grams of proteins in 96g of broccoli and 31 calories.

- ✓ Lean Beef: 22 grams of proteins in 85g of cooked beef and has 184 calories.

✓ Tuna: 39 grams of proteins in 154g of tuna preserved in water and has 179 calories.

✓ Quinoa: 8 grams of proteins in 185g of cooked quinoa and has 222 calories.

✓ Lentils: 18 grams of proteins in 198g of cooked lentils and has 230 calories.

✓ Ezekiel Bread: 4 grams of proteins in one slice and has 80 calories.

✓ Pumpkin Seeds: 5 grams of proteins in 28g and has 125 calories.

✓ Turkey Breast: 24 grams of proteins in 85g of turkey breast and has 146 calories.

✓ Salmon: 19 grams of proteins in 85g of salmon and has 175 calories.

✓ Shrimp: 18 grams of proteins in 85g of shrimp and has 84 calories.

✓ Brussels Sprouts: 2 grams of proteins in 78g of Brussels sprouts and has 28 calories.

✓ Peanuts: 7 grams of proteins in 28g of peanuts and has 159 calories.

When a person wants to follow a healthy diet, another macronutrient they need is carbohydrates. It is one of the three essential ways our body is able to get energy and calories aside from proteins and lipids (or else fats). They basically are the fiber, sugars and starches that can be found in vegetables, fruit, milk products and grain. Carbohydrates are made from oxygen, carbon and hydrogen. They are categorized into two groups according to their chemical structure. Those are:

- ✓ Fast-releasing carbohydrates - also referred to as sugars

- ✓ Slow-releasing carbohydrates - also referred to as polysaccharides

At a molecular level, carbohydrates are only chains of simple sugars. When we eat carbohydrates, our body has to break down the molecule of the carb in separate sugars in order to be absorbed in the intestines so that our bodies can use the nutrition as well as the energy of the carbohydrates. Based on the molecular structure of the carbohydrates, this digestion process can be fast or slow, allowing us to categorize the carbohydrates into the two groups we mentioned before.

In order to measure how fast the carbohydrates are digested in our bodies, we have the glycemic index, or GI, and the glycemic load. The glycemic index is based on how quickly the carbohydrates that are found in food elevate a person's blood sugar levels. When carbohydrates found in food are digested rapidly, they rank high in the glycemic index, when they are digested more slowly, they rank lower in the glycemic index. The glycemic load does not pay attention to the time carbohydrates take to be digested, but it has to do with the level of carbohydrates in the food that the body is able to digest.

Both the glycemic load and glycemic index work to show how a person's body will be able to handle carbohydrates and how it can digest carbs. For example, foods high in glycemic load and glycemic index may elevate a person's blood sugar levels higher than the body itself is able to deal with, thus causing problems in the metabolism and hormones, resulting in the accumulation of body fat.

Some foods that are considered as fast-releasing carbohydrates when tested in laboratories are the following:

- ✓ Short-grain white rice

- ✓ White bread

- ✓ Candy

- ✓ Rice cakes

- ✓ Pretzels

- ✓ Instant mashed potatoes

- ✓ Tapioca pudding

- ✓ Energy bars

- ✓ Cornmeal

- ✓ Sports drinks

- ✓ Soda

- ✓ Dried fruits

- ✓ Fruit leathers

- ✓ Instant oatmeal

- ✓ White jasmine rice

- ✓ Cornmeal mush

Some of the foods that are considered as slow-releasing carbohydrates when they were tested in laboratories include:

- ✓ Whole-wheat tortillas

- ✓ Peanuts

- ✓ Lentils

- ✓ Oats

- ✓ Barley

- ✓ No starchy vegetables

- ✓ Almost all beans

- ✓ Tree nuts

- ✓ Chickpeas

- ✓ Hummus

- ✓ Unsweetened dairy products

- ✓ Starchy pasta

Carbohydrates are essential not only because they are able to provide our bodies with energy but also because they aid in the proper function of the heart, kidneys and the nervous system. Generally, carbs are mentioned as one of the reasons obesity has risen in recent years. However, there are also carbohydrates that are healthy to consume as opposed to processed junk foods that have high levels of sugar. For some people, low-carb diets may be required for health reasons, but overall healthy people are not required to avoid all foods that contain high levels of carbohydrates. The following list contains foods high in carbohydrates that are also very healthy for us:

- ✓ Quinoa: When cooked, quinoa has 21,3% carbs and is also a great source of fiber and proteins.

- ✓ Oats: When raw, oats have 66% carbs out of which almost 11% is fiber. They also contain proteins, at higher levels than other grain.

- ✓ Buckwheat: When raw, buckwheat has 71,5% carbs and when it is cooked it has approximately 20% of carbs. It is also a source of fiber and proteins.

- ✓ Bananas: They contain 23% carbs and are rich in vitamin C and vitamin B6.

- ✓ Sweet Potatoes: When they are cooked they have approximately 18% to 21% carbs. They are also very rich in provitamin A.

- ✓ Beetroots: When they are either raw or cooked beetroots have 8% to 10% of carbs. They are also high in minerals and vitamins.

- ✓ Oranges: They are basically made out of water and have about 11,8% of carbs. Oranges are full of vitamin C.

✓ Blueberries: They are labeled as a superfood since they have large amounts of antioxidants and plant compounds. They are made of about 14,5% of carbs and mainly water.

✓ Grapefruit: It has approximately 9% carbs and is high in minerals and vitamins.

✓ Apples: They have about 13% to 15% carbs and can be used as a source of vitamin C.

✓ Kidney Beans: When they are cooked they have 22,8% of carbs and they are also rich in proteins.

✓ Chickpeas: They are made out of 27,4% of carbs out of which 8% is fiber. They are also rich in minerals and vitamins such as B-vitamins and iron.

As you can see some of the healthiest foods listed here, as well as many more, are rich in carbohydrates and the belief that carbs are not healthy is only a myth. However, they should not be consumed in large amounts, especially refined carbs. Sources of whole food carbs are extremely healthy when consumed in normal amounts.

Lipids are a group of nonpolar molecules that are made out of oxygen, carbon and hydrogen. However, as opposed to carbohydrates, they are are not able to be dissolved in water. They are the building blocks of the function as well as the structure of living cells. Lipids can be found in oils, dairy products, meat, seeds, nuts, butter and processed foods and they can be produced in the liver. They help in the right absorption and digestion of the food we eat and should be an essential part of our diet in appropriate amounts. Their main task is to store energy and, apart from that, they are also able to work as membranes of the cells and protect our organs to help the regulation of our temperature. They are separated into two basic classes:

- ✓ Nonsaponifiable lipids

- ✓ Saponifiable lipids

Nonsaponifiable lipids are defined as the lipids that cannot be broken into smaller molecules through hydrolysis and include waxes, phospholipids, triglycerides as well as sphingolipids. On the other hand, saponifiable lipids are able to go through the process of hydrolysis when they are combined with enzymes, acid or base. In this category, the lipids included are terpenes, steroids and prostaglandins. You will also find the categories of non-polar and polar lipids. In the first group, we will find lipids like triglycerides that are tasked with storing fuel and energy. In the second group, the polar lipids work by forming a barrier that is used in membranes. Polar lipids such as sphingolipids and glycerophospholipids are perfect examples of this task.

Fatty acids are essential components of the lipids. They are carboxylic acids and can be unsaturated or saturated. Generally, unsaturated fat is considered healthier for the body when compared to saturated fat. The difference between those groups is that unsaturated fatty acids have more double bonds than one, as opposed to saturated fatty acids which are full of hydrogen molecules. You will find saturated fat in the following foods:

- ✓ Butter

- ✓ Coconut oil

- ✓ Ice-cream

- ✓ Cheese

- ✓ High-fat parts of meat

- ✓ Pam oil

On the other hand, you will find unsaturated fats in the following foods:

- ✓ Olives

- ✓ Olive oil

- ✓ Avocado

- ✓ Avocado oil

- ✓ Sunflower oil

- ✓ Canola oil

- ✓ Corn oil

- ✓ Salmon

- ✓ Mackerel

- ✓ Peanut oil

- ✓ Peanut butter

- ✓ Almonds

- ✓ Cashews

- ✓ Peanuts

- ✓ Sesame seeds

In other words, lipids are fats and, for this reason, many people believe they should avoid altogether foods that are high in fat due to the fact that those foods will, in turn, make them fat. However, the truth is that the human body needs fat since it is perfect for storing energy and thus turning into source of fuel for us. Diets emphasize on lipids, or else fats, along with proteins and carbohydrates, especially fats that come from food containing omega-6 and omega-3. The key for the lipids to not make you fat, as many people believe, is moderation. Let us see which foods that are high in fat are extremely healthy for us:

- ✓ Avocados: They contain 77% of fat and are a perfect source of potassium since they have 40% more potassium than even bananas. They are also rich in fiber and are able to lower triglycerides and LDL cholesterol.

- ✓ Cheese: Even though it is high in fat, cheese can work as a rich source of vitamin B12, calcium, selenium and phosphorus since in order to make one slice of cheese you need one whole cup of milk.

- ✓ Dark Chocolate: In terms of fat it contains 65% of calories, but is rich in iron, manganese, magnesium and copper. It is also full of antioxidants, to the extent that it beats blueberries.

- ✓ Whole eggs: Generally, they were believed to be unhealthy due to the fact that the yolks were high in fat and cholesterol. Specifically, one egg has 212 mg of cholesterol and 62% of the calories come from fat. However, research has shown that in most people the cholesterol in eggs does not affect the cholesterol in the blood. Whole eggs are full in minerals and vitamins and in fact, include a small amount of almost every nutrient we need.

- ✓ Fatty Fish: They refer to fish such as trout, sardines, salmon, herring and mackerel. These fish are extremely healthy since they are rich in omega-3 fatty acids and proteins.

- ✓ Nuts: They contain high amounts of fibers, fats, and vitamin E as well as magnesium. According to research, people who include nuts in their diet have the tendency to be healthier and with a lower risk of some diseases. Some of those include walnuts, almonds and macadamia.

- ✓ Chia Seeds: They may not be considered as food filled with fats but there are 9 grams of fat in 28gr of chia seeds. More specifically, in terms of calories, chia seeds contain 80% of fat. Most of the fats in them are healthy omega-3 fatty acids that are great for the heart.

- ✓ Extra Virgin Olive Oil: The vast majority of experts agree that extra virgin olive oil is extremely healthy and is an essential part of the Mediterranean diet that has many benefits as shown many times in the past. This oil is rich in vitamins K and E as well as in strong antioxidants.

✓ Coconut oil and Coconuts: They are rich and are the main source of saturated fat all over the world. More specifically 90% of their fatty acids are saturated. The types of fats coconut oil and coconuts have, are extremely helpful for people who have Alzheimer's.

✓ Full-Fat Yogurt: It is extremely healthy like other dairy products that are high in fat and, in addition, it is rich in probiotic bacteria that can be very beneficial for a person to stay healthy.

Last but not least, on the list of macronutrients is one element that we must also take in large amounts on a daily basis, water. It is a true fact that our adult bodies are made of a total of 60% of water. More specifically, the heart and brain are made up of 73% of water and our lungs are made approximately of 83% of water. To stress the importance of water even more, the skin has 64% of water and the kidneys, as well as muscles, contain 79% of water. Also, our bones contain up to 31% of water. Water exists in nearly everything we eat and drink every day with research showing that an adult takes in about two liters of water each day from his or her drink and food.

It is a fact that a person will be able to survive without water for only three days and this shows its importance for the human body. It has many functions and some of them include it being an essential nutrient to every cell in our bodies since it also works as a building material. Water is also able to regulate the temperature in our bodies through respiration and sweating. In addition to this, the proteins and carbohydrates, after they are metabolized, are transported in the bloodstream through water. It is used to lubricate the joints, it creates the saliva, and it helps us flush waste out of our bodies, mainly through urination.

For these reasons, if you are not hydrated through the day your brain function, as well as your energy levels, will drop according to many studies. When we increase the amount of water we drink every day there are several health benefits. More specifically an increased amount of water intake will help you deal with:

- ✓ Cancer

- ✓ Constipation

- ✓ Acne

- ✓ Kidney stones

- ✓ Skin hydration

Our bodies have an amazing system of their own to warn you when your water reserves are running low and this is called thirst. Trust your body and drink plenty of water even when you think you are not thirsty enough to get out of your warm bed or while watching an amazing movie.

Moving on, as micronutrients we consider those nutrients that can be found in smaller amounts in our bodies, but this does not mean that they are not essential for the body to function properly. In the category of micronutrients, we will find all the essential vitamins and minerals and there are sixteen minerals and thirteen vitamins to consider. One difference between lipids, carbohydrates, proteins and micronutrients is that the last ones are not used directly for the purpose of creating energy. Micronutrients will be able to help in the process of making energy by being a part of enzymes. Enzymes are considered proteins that bring about chemical reactions in our bodies and are part of its functions.

There are thirteen essential vitamins that are defined as organic compounds. In other words, they are carbon-based and can be further categorized as being fat-soluble or water-soluble. The fat-soluble vitamins are K, D, A and E and are stored in the fatty tissues of the body. Those vitamins that are water-soluble include vitamin C and every B vitamins that are the following:

- ✓ Thiamine (Vitamin B1)

- ✓ Riboflavin (Vitamin B2)

- ✓ Niacin (Vitamin B3)

- ✓ Pantothenic acid (Vitamin B5)

- ✓ Pyroxidine (Vitamin B6)

- ✓ Biotin (Vitamin B7)

- ✓ Folate (Vitamin B9)

- ✓ Cobalamin (Vitamin B12)

Water-soluble vitamins need to be renewed often since they are taken out of the body through urine. The only water-soluble vitamin that is not taken out of the body and is instead stored in the liver is the vitamin B12. In order for a person to have enough of all the 13 essential vitamins in their body, they have to obtain them through a balanced diet. Let us see in more detail why a person needs to have those vitamins in the appropriate amounts and the best source of food for each vitamin.

Vitamin A:

It is an integral part in the development and growth of the cells. This vitamin will also help us have healthy nails, skin, glands, hair, gums, teeth and bones. It is also capable of preventing night blindness and it may aid in the prevention of lung cancer. The best source of food for vitamin A is cold-water fish such as salmon, dairy products, and egg yolks.

Vitamin D:

This vitamin will help us in the absorption of calcium and in extension it aids in building and maintaining strong teeth and bones. The best source of vitamin D is milk, rice or soy beverages, oil from fish liver, egg yolks, exposure to the sun and fatty fish.

Vitamin E:

This vitamin is tasked with the protection of fatty acids and the maintenance of the red blood cells as well as the maintenance of muscles. It is also a crucial antioxidant and you will be able to find this vitamin in vegetable oils, mayonnaise, eggs, margarine, cereals, seeds and nuts.

Vitamin K:

For proper blood-clotting, vitamin K is the key and, for this reason, it is an essential vitamin for our bodies. The main sources for vitamin K are broccoli, liver, spinach and green leafy vegetables.

Vitamin C - Ascorbic Acid:

This vitamin is able to provide your blood vessel walls with strength and to enhance the absorption of iron as well as the healing of various wounds. It will also help in preventing atherosclerosis and will support your immune system. Vitamin C is another essential antioxidant and can be found in melons, citrus fruits, peppers, berries, potatoes and broccoli.

Thiamine - Vitamin B1:

This vitamin is essential in keeping your metabolism healthy and preserves a normal appetite, nerve function and digestion. You will be able to find Vitamin B1 in abundance in legumes, cereals, nuts, grains, seeds and pork.

Riboflavin - Vitamin B2:

This vitamin is important in the metabolism of energy and will also be able to help in the function of the adrenal gland; it will support your normal vision and keep your skin healthy. You will find this vitamin in abundance in the following sources, lean meat, cereals, dairy products, grain, raw mushrooms, rice and soy.

Niacin - Vitamin B3:

This is another vitamin with an essential function for the body since it is used to metabolize the energy in our bodies and enhance our normal growth. When this vitamin is taken in high amounts, it can also lower cholesterol. You will be able to find this vitamin in abundance in poultry, milk, lean meats, legumes, cereals, bread, seafood and eggs.

Pantothenic Acid - Vitamin B5:

This vitamin can be found easily and is also essential for bodily functions. It will help the metabolism of energy and keep the blood sugar at normal levels. As we said it is relatively easy to find since it is an ingredient in almost all foods.

Pyridoxine - Vitamin B6:

In order to be healthy, this vitamin is also an essential one. It will aid in the metabolism of proteins and carbohydrates, and will also help in the release of our energy. It will also help the body in the formation of red blood cells and will also play an important role in the correct function of the nerves. You will find this vitamin in abundance in grain, meat, cereals, fish, poultry, bananas, potatoes, green leafy vegetables and soybeans.

Biotin - Vitamin B7:

This vitamin is important in maintaining your metabolism at a healthy level. This vitamin will be found in soybeans, yeast, egg yolks, nuts and soybeans.

Folate - Vitamin B9:

This vitamin is very important, especially for women who are pregnant. This is the case because vitamin B9 is essential in the formation of RNA, DNA, red blood cells and in synthesizing some particular amino acids. It is also capable of helping pregnant women in the prevention of birth defects. This vitamin can be found in abundance in yeast, asparagus, liver, orange juice, leafy green vegetables, legumes, flour and avocados.

Cobalamin - Vitamin B12:

This vitamin is also essential because it will help in the formation of RNA, DNA, red blood cells as well as myelin for the nerve fiber. You will be able to find this vitamin in all the animal products.

As we can conclude from the above analysis, severe deficiencies of those vitamins can, in turn, cause severe problems to our health. Let us take for example the disease of pellagra which is a result of the deficiency of niacin and was a common occurrence in certain parts of America during the early years of the twentieth century. The most common symptoms of this disease were left in history with the name "4D's" and stand for dermatitis, diarrhea, dementia and last death. The solution to this disease came when scientists discovered that balanced diets relieved the symptoms of pellagra.

Moving on to minerals, they are defined as an inorganic substance that is solid and can occur naturally. They can also be divided into two categories based on the amount we need to take. The truth is that our bodies need many minerals and those are named essential minerals. Those essential minerals are then separated into the two categories of macrominerals and microminerals (or else trace minerals).

These two categories have the same level of importance to us with the only difference being the fact that we need a smaller amount of trace minerals than macrominerals. However, keep in mind that this distinction is based on the amount we need, not their importance. In other words, just because we need fewer amounts of trace minerals, this doesn't mean that they are not as important as macrominerals.

A balanced diet will give us all the essential minerals, no matter the category they fall in. Generally, minerals have regulatory, metabolic and structural capabilities. A common example of the structural capabilities of minerals is the construction of teeth and bones. They can also synthesize hormones, relax the muscles of the body and transmit the nerve impulses, as well as protect the organism from free radicals that can be very harmful. Let us see in more detail the minerals in each group, their effects on the body as well as the foods we will be able to find them in.

<u>Macrominerals</u>:

Sodium:

This macromineral is essential for the body to balance its fluids, for the contraction of the muscles and for the transmission of the nerves. You will be able to find it in soy sauce and table salt, as well as in larger amounts in all the processed foods. In smaller amounts, it exists in vegetables, milk, bread and in unprocessed meats.

Chloride:

This mineral is essential for the production of stomach acid as well as for the body to balance its fluids. You will find it in larger amounts in all processed foods, table salt and soy sauce. In smaller amounts, it exists in vegetables, milk, meat and bread.

Potassium:

This macromineral is also important for the body to balance its fluids, the transmission of nerves, and the contraction of the muscles. Some rich sources of potassium are meat, milk, legumes, fresh vegetables, fresh fruits and whole grain.

Calcium:

This macromineral is extremely important for our organism since it is able to maintain healthy teeth and bones as well as to aid in the relaxation and contraction of the muscles. It is also essential for the functions of the nerves, the regulation of blood pressure, blood clotting and the overall health of our immune system. You will find it abundantly in milk products, milk, salmon, fortified tofu, sardines and all canned fish that have bones, fortified soy milk, mustard greens, legumes and broccoli.

Phosphorus:

This is another mineral that is very important due to the fact that it also helps us to maintain healthy teeth and bones and is found in every cell. Phosphorus is also present in the body's system that keeps the acid-base balance. You will find it in all processed foods, fish, meat, poultry and eggs.

Magnesium:

This mineral is always present in our bones and is very important for the production of proteins, the transmission of nerves, the overall health of our immune system and for the contraction of our muscles. Rich sources of magnesium are seeds and nuts as well as leafy green vegetables, chocolate, legumes and artichokes.

Sulfur:

You will be able to find this macromineral in protein molecules and is present in foods such as legumes, fish, nuts, meats, milk and poultry.

Microminerals:

Iron:

This mineral is categorized as a micromineral even though the amount of iron the body needs is relatively higher than that of the other microminerals we will analyze shortly. Iron is a part of the molecule hemoglobin and can be located in the red blood cells that carry oxygen throughout the body. Iron is essential in energy metabolism and can be found in large amounts in organ and red meat, legumes, fish, shellfish, dried fruits, egg yolks, poultry, leafy green vegetables, cereals, bread as well as fortified cereals.

Zinc:

This micromineral is a component of various enzymes and is essential for the production of genetic material and protein. It helps us in the perception of taste, in the healthy development of a fetus, in the healing of wounds, in the appropriate production of sperm, in the overall health of our immune system, in growing at a healthy pace and in sexual maturity. This mineral is mainly found in poultry, meat, leaved whole grain, fish and vegetables.

Iodine:

This mineral is located in the thyroid hormone which aids us in the regulation of healthy growth, metabolism and development. You will find this micromineral in foods that grow in rich with iodine soil, seafood, bread, salt and dairy products.

Selenium:

This mineral is an antioxidant and is found in grain, meats and seafood.

Copper:

This micromineral is a component of various enzymes and is essential in the metabolism of iron. You will find it in nuts, legumes, seeds, organ meat, whole grain and in drinking water.

Fluoride:

Even though this mineral is categorized as a micromineral, it is essential in the formation of teeth and bones and it aids in the prevention of the decay of our teeth. You will find it in the water we drink, almost all teas and fish.

Chromium:

This mineral cooperates at a high level with insulin in order to regulate the levels of the sugar in our blood. You will find it in brewer's yeast, nuts, unrefined foods and cheese.

Molybdenum:

This micromineral is a component of several enzymes and you will be able to find it in grain, bread, legumes, leafy green vegetables, liver and milk.

Everything we have analyzed so far needs to be added to your diet in order for you to be able to call it "balanced" and achieve your optimal health no matter the source of food you choose to take those nutrients from. We have mentioned the meat sources in order for this chapter to work as a complete guide on what balanced diets should contain, but it is a fact that more and more people nowadays choose to abandon some or all meat, and meat products, altogether.

The Levels of Vegetarianism

Research has shown that over 18% of the world population has chosen to follow a different type of diet that is called vegetarianism. Vegetarianism is about abstention from the consumption of meat as well as from all the different products of animal slaughter. However, there are various levels of this practice based on how a person defines meat. Before we move on with our analysis of these levels, we will present the different food groups in order for you to get a better grasp of vegetarianism and its levels.

Foods are generally separated into five different categories based on the common amounts of essential nutrients they provide us with. For example, the food group of fruit provides a considerable amount of vitamins and, more specifically, a considerable amount of vitamin C. Let us take a closer look at each group respectively.

Group One: Legumes/Beans and Vegetables:

Research has shown that if we consume vegetables everyday, we are less in danger of having coronary heart disease. Also, we are less at risk of gaining weight and going through a stroke by consuming vegetables, especially the colorful ones. Vegetables, along with beans and legumes, are low in kilojoules and they are a proper source of vitamins including folate and vitamin C. They are also a source of magnesium, minerals, dietary fiber and they are filled with nutrients.

Generally, vegetables are derived from different parts of a plant such as the roots, flowers, leaves, seeds, shoots, tubers and stems. Legumes derive from the seeds of a plant and are consumed as green beans and peas when in their immature form and as dried beans, chickpeas, peas and lentils when in their mature form. We have different groups of vegetables based on the nutrients they are able to provide. More specifically, those groups include:

<u>Root - Tubular - Bulb Vegetables</u>:

- ✓ Cassava
- ✓ Taro
- ✓ Potato
- ✓ Sweet Potato
- ✓ Carrots
- ✓ Onions
- ✓ Garlic
- ✓ Beetroot
- ✓ Shallots
- ✓ Shoots
- ✓ Turnip
- ✓ Bamboo

✓ Swede

Dark Green or else Cruciferous - Brassica:

✓ Brussels sprouts

✓ Cabbage

✓ Broccoli

✓ Bok Choy

✓ Cauliflower

✓ Kale

✓ Silverbeet

✓ Snow Peas

✓ Lettuce

✓ Spinach

Legumes - Beans

✓ Soybeans

✓ Chickpeas

✓ Red kidney beans

- ✓ Lima beans

- ✓ Lentils

- ✓ Cannellini beans

- ✓ Split peas

- ✓ Tofu

<u>More Vegetables</u>:

- ✓ Sprouts

- ✓ Squash

- ✓ Tomato

- ✓ Zucchini

- ✓ Celery

- ✓ Capsicum

- ✓ Mushrooms

- ✓ Avocado

- ✓ Eggplant

- ✓ Okra

- ✓ Green beans

- ✓ Pumpkin

- ✓ Green peas

- ✓ Celery

<u>Group Two: Fruit</u>

Many people do not eat much fruit but drink many fruit juices. Whole fruits are even better to consume since fruit juices have the potential to be low in dietary fiber, damage your teeth, but can also be high in kilojoules, or else energy. For you to get the best quality of fruit, you should choose the ones which are appropriate for each season of the year and this way you will also have a wide range of fruit added to your diet. As is the case with the vegetable group, opting for fruit of different colors will offer you a wider range of nutrients, thus making you healthier. Let us see the different food categories and some of the fruit associated with them:

<u>Pome Fruit</u>:

- ✓ Medlar

- ✓ Apple

- ✓ Loquat

- ✓ Chokeberry

- ✓ Pear

- ✓ Rosehip

- ✓ Saskatoon Berry

- ✓ Rowan

- ✓ Quince

- ✓ Shipova

Citrus Fruit:

- ✓ Grapefruit

- ✓ Lemon

- ✓ Lime

- ✓ Mandarin orange

- ✓ Tangerines

- ✓ Sweet oranges

- ✓ Bergamot

- ✓ Kumquat

- ✓ Kinnow

- ✓ Ponderosa lemon

✓ Satsuma

✓ Sudachi

✓ Tangelo

Stone Fruit

✓ Peaches

✓ Plums

✓ Apricots

✓ Nectarines

✓ Apricots

✓ Blackberries

✓ Apriums

✓ Pluots

✓ Mulberries

✓ Cherries

✓ Green almonds

✓ Mangoes

✓ Lychees

- ✓ Coconut

- ✓ Olives

- ✓ Dates

Tropical Fruit

- ✓ Banana

- ✓ Breadfruit

- ✓ Cherimoya

- ✓ Mango

- ✓ Paw paw

- ✓ Pineapple

- ✓ Melons

Other Fruit

- ✓ Berries

- ✓ Grapes

- ✓ Passionfruit

Group Three: Grain - Cereals Group

As grain food, we define all the foods that are made mostly out of rice, wheat, quinoa, corn, barley, rye, millet, and oats. Grain give us the opportunity to be cooked in order for us to consume them, made into flour and create different types of cereal foods such as pasta, noodles and bread or even create cereals for breakfast. The grain - cereal foods can be further divided into four essential categories. Those are:

Bread:

- ✓ Wholegrain

- ✓ Rye

- ✓ Lavash

- ✓ Crispbreads

- ✓ White

- ✓ Wholemeal

- ✓ Pita

- ✓ Naan

- ✓ Focaccia

Breakfast Cereals:

- ✓ High fibre - Wholegrain

✓ Ready to eat

✓ Porridge

✓ Wholewheat

✓ Muesli

✓ Oats

✓ Biscuits

<u>Grains</u>:

✓ Barley

✓ Rice

✓ Corn

✓ Buckwheat

✓ Polenta

✓ Spelt

✓ Sorghum

✓ Millet

✓ Triticale

✓ Rye

✓ Semolina

✓ Quinoa

<u>Others Include</u>:

✓ Noodles

✓ Crumpet

✓ Pasta

✓ English muffin

✓ Couscous

✓ Flour

✓ Popcorn

When we talk about wholegrain cereal, we mean the food that has three covers of grain. Those will have more minerals, antioxidants, vitamins and fiber than other cereals that are refined, as is the case with white bread, due to the fact that many essential nutrients that are located on the outer cover of the grain are gone because of the processing it undergoes. Wholegrain foods are extremely essential to vegetarian diets since they are an important source of zinc and iron.

Also, when we mention refined grain, such as white flour, we talk about the food that has the germ and bran layers taken away. Because of this process, much of the vitamins, fiber, phytochemical and minerals is gone. Even though in some cases some of the minerals and vitamins are able to be added again as it happens with white bread, it is not the same and, most of the time, the full benefits are lost completely. Keep in mind that phytochemicals, which are very beneficial for our overall health as is shown by many studies, cannot be placed back again.

The various nutrients given by grain include proteins, the B vitamins thiamin, niacin, folate, zinc, vitamin E, phosphorus, magnesium and carbohydrates. Also, wholegrain and cereal foods are able to lessen the chances of having coronary heart disease, diverticular disease, diabetes and colon cancer. In addition to this, high fibre whole grain cereals will help you maintain your digestive system at healthy levels and prevent constipation. Not to mention that high fiber foods like wholegrain cereals and bread are recommended in many diets for the purpose of weight loss since they take more time to digest and make you feel full, which in turn keeps you from overeating. Last but not least, whole grains have polyunsaturated fatty acids which are very beneficial for our health and are low in saturated fat.

<u>Group Four: Lean Meat and Eggs, Poultry, Tofu, Fish, Nuts, Seeds, and Legumes - Beans</u>

The foods that belong to this group are generally considered rich in proteins. They also provide us with many nutrients including zinc, iodine, vitamins - more importantly B12 - fatty acids and iron. Iron is extremely important for young girls, menstruating women, pregnant women, as well as endurance athletes. According to experts, the zinc and iron found in animal foods can be absorbed in an easier way than those found in plant foods like seeds, legumes - beans, and nuts, but the vitamin C that is present in vegetables and fruit will aid in absorbing the iron from any food that does not come from animals.

Legumes are able to offer us a lot of the nutrients we will find in fish, lean meats, eggs and poultry and, for this reason, they are placed in this group too aside from the food group of vegetables. Legumes are extremely important in vegan diets for the people to absorb enough nutrients that are found in this group and are based on meat. The foods of this group can be separated into 6 further categories. Those are:

<u>Lean meat</u>:

- ✓ Lamb

- ✓ Pork

- ✓ Beef

- ✓ Veal

- ✓ Kangaroo

- ✓ Lean sausages

Poultry:

- ✓ Turkey

- ✓ Emu

- ✓ Chicken

- ✓ Duck

- ✓ Bush Birds

- ✓ Goose

Seafood and Fish:

- ✓ Prawns

- ✓ Lobster

- ✓ Fish

- ✓ Crab

- ✓ Mussels

- ✓ Scallops

✓ Clams

✓ Oysters

<u>Eggs</u>:

✓ Duck eggs

✓ Chicken eggs

<u>Seeds and Nuts</u>:

✓ Pine nuts

✓ Macadamia

✓ Almonds

✓ Hazelnut

✓ Peanuts

✓ Cashew

✓ Pumpkin seeds

✓ Sunflower seeds

✓ Nut Spreads

✓ Sesame seeds

- ✓ Brazil nuts

<u>Legumes - Beans</u>:

- ✓ Chickpeas

- ✓ Tofu

- ✓ Lentils

- ✓ Split peas

- ✓ All beans

For the diets that include no meat but allow milk products, nuts, seeds, eggs and legumes a person will be able to get all the main nutrients for staying healthy. However, vitamin B12 can be taken only from animal products and for diets that restrict all animal products and meat, a supplement may be needed.

Group Five: Milk, Yogurt, Cheese and/or Alternative

This group includes milk, yogurt, cheese and their alternatives. We can find a wide range of yogurt and milk products that have different levels of fat. You can find milk that is evaporated, fresh, dried or with a long life (or else UHT). Also, cheese has high amounts of kilojoules, salt and saturated fat, but there are also cheeses that have fewer amounts of salt and fat. Let us see which foods are included in this category:

<u>Milk</u>:

- ✓ Plain milk
- ✓ Flavored milk
- ✓ All reduced-fat milk
- ✓ Full cream milk
- ✓ Long-life milk
- ✓ Soy beverages
- ✓ Powdered milk
- ✓ Evaporated milk

<u>Yogurt</u>:

- ✓ Plain yogurt
- ✓ Flavored yogurt
- ✓ Reduced-fat yogurt
- ✓ Full cream yogurt
- ✓ Soy yogurt

<u>Cheese</u>:

- ✓ All hard cheese

- ✓ Full fat cheese

- ✓ Reduced-fat cheese

- ✓ Red Leicester

- ✓ Edam

- ✓ Gouda Soy cheese

- ✓ Gloucester

Yogurt, milk and cheese are able to offer us calcium in a form that can be absorbed easily by our bodies. They are also rich in various nutrients such as iodine, vitamin D, vitamin A, vitamin B12, zinc and proteins.

Now that we have a full understanding of the different food groups as well as the various nutrients they can offer us, let us move on to the main part of this chapter which is analyzing the different levels of vegetarianism. As we have mentioned, the levels of vegetarianism have to do with which foods you want to include in your diet and which foods you would like to exclude.

However, one thing is common in all the levels and that is the fact that no meat is allowed except in some specific levels where animal flesh or fish is "allowed" to be eaten. You will meet on many occasions the distinction between a vegetarian and a vegan. The truth is that they are both levels, or else types, of the vegetarian diet, so you shouldn't be confused. Let us start with the presentation of the various levels of vegetarianism.

Level 1: Flexitarian or else Semi-Vegetarian

People who are on this level are not considered by many vegetarians as "true vegetarians" due to the fact that the term "Flexitarian" was created to describe all those who follow mostly the vegetarian diet but consume meat occasionally. Those people who call themselves semi-vegetarian or flexitarian do not consume meat most commonly for health reasons, while others eat organic or free-range animal products and animals mainly for environmental reasons.

However, it is a fact that vegetarians do not eat meat and a semi-vegetarian or flexitarian is not a true vegetarian. It is also a fact that almost all true vegetarians do not recognize the use of this term. This level was created mostly at first to describe the people who are in the process of cutting meat from their diets and are not able to do so completely from the moment they decided to be vegetarians.

Also, there is not a clear definition of how often a flexitarian eats meat. It is only used to describe a general situation when a person follows mostly the diet of vegetarians but eats meat on several occasions. Whether this person eats meat once a day or once a year is left completely up to him or her. This is also another reason why this term is resented by many true vegetarians since they claim that there is no such thing as almost vegetarian in the same way that there is no such thing as being almost pregnant. Vegetarians and meat do not go together.

No matter the arguments, this term and level show an important step in the right direction for saving the environment, the animals and developing our health and, based on the premise that this person will strive to achieve the goal of vegetarianism, it should be a great thing.

Level 2: Pescatarian or else Pescetarian

The word pescatarian or pescetarian usually refers to people who do not eat meat at all or animal flesh with one exception: fish. Essentially, this person keeps up with the vegetarian diet but adds fish or other seafood like clams, lobster, shrimps and crabs. To put it simply, a person who calls himself or herself pescatarian eats fish and does not eat any kind of meat such as steak, pork, chicken or anything else that has to do with meat, only seafood and fish aside from the mainly vegetarian foods including vegetables, tofu, grain, beans, dairy and fruit.

The same problem applies here as in the case of the flexitarians. A pescatarian is not a vegetarian and this type of diet exists for mainly health reasons as is the case with high cholesterol and people who wish to eliminate meat while still getting proteins from a common source; another reason can be a build-up towards a completely vegetarian diet.

In the second case, some people may have been able to cut off meat but not fish or seafood and will do so as time passes. It is a fact that some people may like more fish and seafood over a steak while other people like more meat than fish and seafood. In both situations, they choose to cut off completely their favorite option in stages until they are able to not consume it anymore.

There are also people who follow this type of diet because they think that a controlled consumption of fish oils or fish, which have high levels of Omega-3 fatty acids, is essential for better health, even though there are alternatives for vegetarians like hemp foods or flaxseed oil.

If someone wants to adopt a vegetarian diet, but still thinks that fish is an essential source for protein, he or she should know that this should not be the only reason for adopting a pescatarian diet. We can find many sources of proteins that have nothing to do with meat or fish such as beans, nuts, and lentils. It has been proven that a person is able to follow through a diet that is rich in protein without having to eat fish or meat.

Even though a pescatarian is not considered a vegetarian because the vegetarian diet forbids the consumption of all animals, and fish are animals, it is included as a level of vegetarianism when it is based on the premise that the said person is going to eventually stop any consumption of fish or seafood.

<u>Level 3: Lacto or Ovo Vegetarian</u>

This type of vegetarian is the most common in North America. The people that identify themselves as Lacto and Ovo vegetarians do not eat fish, poultry, beef, insects, pork, animal flesh, or shellfish but they do eat eggs and dairy products. The word Lacto stems from the Latin word for milk and Ovo stands for egg. More particularly a Lacto vegetarian is someone who is a vegetarian and does not consume eggs but chooses to consume dairy products. There are a lot of Hindu vegetarians that fall in this type of diet of not eating eggs but keep consuming dairy products mainly for religious reasons.

The term Ovo vegetarian is used to describe people who have excluded meat from their diet as well as dairy products but keep eating eggs. One common reason for vegetarians to choose this type of diet is that they are lactose intolerant. In this level, there are also problems that have to do with a debate on whether Lacto and Ovo vegetarians are true vegetarians. Some people maintain that eggs should be included in a vegetarian diet and others, especially in the United Kingdom, maintain that particular types of cheese should be excluded from a vegetarian diet too.

<u>Level 4: Vegan</u>

The term "vegan" is used to describe both a person that has adopted the vegan way of eating and the vegan diet as a whole. Veganism is described as a certain type of vegetarian diet and is based on the exclusion of eggs, meat, dairy products and every other product or food that has been derived from animals. This also means excluding foods that had been produced by using animal products like certain wines and refined white sugar. There are many wines as well as beers that have been refined with the usage of a product that is named isinglass. This product is produced from fish and may even be filtered with bone char.

The debate that exists here has to do with whether some particular foods like honey should be included in a vegan diet. In this case, each person will choose individually if those foods should be consumed or not.

Veganism though does not linger only on food. For example, vegans will avoid using all products that have been tested on animals and will not buy any products that are derived from animals and are not food such as wool, leather, and fur.

A vegan diet includes all beans, fruit, legumes, and vegetables as well as nearly all the foods that can be produced through a combination of those foods. Also, there are vegan versions of many popular foods such as vegan ice-cream, hot dogs, cheese, vegan mayonnaise, non-dairy yogurt, and vegan burgers as well as other substitutes for meat. Some other foods that have been linked with veganism are non-dairy milk substitutes, soy milk, and tofu.

Vegans are allowed to eat everyday foods such as vegetarian Thai curry which is created from coconut milk and a vegetarian burrito that excludes sour cream. Foods like cheese, green salad, peanut butter, spaghetti, cornbread, salsa, and chips are also included in the vegan diet. Vegans are considered by many people as the last level of veganism, the ultimate goal of all other levels and as the true vegetarians of the world that have nothing to do with anything that includes animal usage and of course cruelty.

Those were the levels of vegetarianism with the last one being the target of many people who wish, for various reasons, to indulge in a completely different lifestyle from what they have been used to before. However, maybe the most surprising thing for some is the growing number of athletes that have adopted this lifestyle, a fact that has been observed to happen in recent years. We use the word surprising because there probably is an educational gap where veganism is concerned and more specifically the reasons people, as well as athletes, choose to make this important turn and generally on the vegan philosophy.

This educational gap is what we aim to tackle in the next chapter where we will present the different reasons that help people make the final decision and change their lives for the better while maintaining a healthy lifestyle based on the vegan philosophy.

The Reasons to Become Vegan

Many people who meet a person that follows a vegan diet will most probably ask "What can you eat?" The truth is that a person who follows a vegan diet can eat everything they want. However, vegans choose to not eat particular things. Veganism is more than just food, it has to do with a particular philosophy, mindset, and ethics.

November the 1st is the World Vegan day where people who don't eat meat, eggs, cheese, whey, mayonnaise, gelatin, or anything that is derived from or includes animals are celebrated. This celebration was established in 1994 and is not just about the people who aid in the development of a world that is free from animal cruelty, but for the animals themselves too. In fact, veganism did not start in 1994 but can actually be traced back to the ancient eastern Mediterranean and Indian societies.

The practice of vegetarianism was mentioned for the first time by the Greek mathematician and philosopher Pythagoras of Samos and is dated around 500 BCE. Pythagoras was not only devoted to the creation of his theorem about right triangles; he also promoted the benevolence between all species and he included humans too. The followers of Hinduism, Jainism, and Buddhism also supported vegetarianism and believed that it was wrong for humans to inflict any kind of pain on other animals.

During the 18th century, Jeremy Bentham who was a utilitarian philosopher advocated his strong opinions that the suffering of animals was as serious as the suffering of humans. He also compared the belief of human superiority to racism. In 1847 the first vegetarian society was formed in England and after three years the American Vegetarian Society was co-founded by Rev. Sylvester Graham who had created the Graham crackers. Rev. Sylvester Graham was also a Presbyterian minister and the people who followed him were called Grahamites. They followed his instructions that helped them lead a moral life including the following rules: abstinence, frequent bathing, vegetarianism, and temperance.

In November 1944 Donald Watson, who was a British woodworker, declared that due to the fact that vegetarians consumed eggs and dairy products, he would invent a new idea that would be called "vegan" and this term would be appropriate to describe the people that were not eating neither eggs nor dairy products. The year prior to Watson's declaration, 40% of the cows that resided in England were diagnosed with tuberculosis and he was able to use this fact to further establish his way of thinking, maintaining that the lifestyle vegans followed protected humans from food that was tainted. By the time Watson perished at the age of 95 years old in 2005, the people that followed the vegan lifestyle reached 250,000 in Britain and in the United States, the number reached 2 million people.

Even though the vegan diet was defined from the start, the term vegan lacked a complete definition and this was achieved in 1949 when Leslie J Cross suggested the existence of this problem and offered the following definition: "[t]he principle of the emancipation of animals from exploitation by man" which was later expanded as "to seek an end to the use of animals by man for food, commodities, work, hunting, vivisection,

57

and by all other uses involving exploitation of animal life by man". A full definition of the vegan way of life came in use in 1988 having endured little change over the years. This definition is the following one:

" […] a philosophy and way of living which seeks to exclude—as far as is possible and practicable—all forms of exploitation of, and cruelty to, animals for food, clothing or any other purpose; and by extension, promotes the development and use of animal-free alternatives for the benefit of humans, animals, and the environment. In dietary terms, it denotes the practice of dispensing with all products derived wholly or partly from animals."

According to The Vegan Society, "Veganism is a way of living which seeks to exclude, as far as is possible and practicable, all forms of exploitation of, and cruelty to, animals for food, clothing or any other purpose". Generally, all vegans follow a diet based on plants and exclude all animal foods like meat including insects, fish, eggs, honey, shellfish, dairy, and eggs as well as not using materials and products that are derived from animals or have been tested on them. Also, vegans avoid all places that are using animals for entertainment reasons.

It is a fact that veganism is a philosophy that has to do with life and thus it has its main principles as well as values. All vegans view life as something that needs to be respected, treasured, and revered. Life applies to all living things and thus animals are not an enemy that has to be put down or used for fun, fabric, or food. Animals were not placed on Earth only to be used by humans.

Vegans do not believe that they are the masters or owners of the natural world, they are a part of the world that will try to protect all species. Also, there are no overpopulated or expendable species that need to be destroyed or hurt. No species or life-forms need to justify their existence or to be forced to be placed in the need for protection because they are in danger of being extinct due to human exploitation by using them as food or test subjects for medicine.

All life is legitimate and veganism rejects any type of hierarchy of species or suffering even to creatures that are deemed to have "primitive nervous systems". Killing those creatures because a distinction was created between them and creatures with "highly developed nervous systems" is not acceptable and every life is of equal value, be it a crayfish, a cockroach, a cow, a carp, a clam, a child, or a chicken. Also, to veganism, peace and gentleness should not be achieved through conflict, violence, and contention and harmony should be accrued through strife.

The ideals of vegans encompass much more than a diet that excludes animal products and defends the rights of animals with fervor. Veganism does not accept the banishment of any sentient being, be it human or animal, from its compassion and benevolence. Veganism does not promote the saving of animals at the expense of humans by treating them with contempt. Vegans love both animals and humans to the same extent and treating humans with disgrace and disrespect is a serious contradiction to the principles of the vegan philosophy.

The most important value of veganism is the fact that life should be respected and treated with compassion, thus placing aside any individual interests that have to do with comfort, cuisine, custom, or convenience. Everything is connected and linked to something else and our actions are connected to something else too. Actions have repercussions for the world we live in whether this repercussion is immediately seen or is happening far away from us and we are not able to see it.

The goal of veganism is to create a world where people are close and the fortune, as well as the fate of every creature on this planet, is not based on generosity or judgment of one species. This will be achieved through the commitment of the people to the vegan philosophy and its values and through exercising mindfulness. All vegans try to be aware, concerned, and thoughtful about the impact of their choices, decisions, and actions. Vegans have confidence and are committed to their ethics, are at peace with themselves, and have a sense of fulfillment and purpose.

Many people make the difference and adopt this lifestyle as well as the values of veganism. Even athletes, whose needs in a balanced diet differ from the ones of an average person, make this change, showing to everyone that a vegan diet and lifestyle apply to every person. Venus Williams, tennis champion, to Lewis Hamilton from Formula 1's and Derrick Morgan the NFL's Tennessee Titans are some examples that prove the boosting power of having a diet based on plants, their performance has not changed a bit from excluding meat as well as products coming from animals. Why more and more athletes make this change, however? There are many reasons that answer this pressing question.

Everyone and even athletes who are at the peak of their health are at risk of having a heart disease. Based on a study that had been conducted on runners and endurance cyclists, it was found that 44 percent of them had coronary plaques. By following a diet based on plants the hearts of athletes remain at their healthiest by reversing plaque, reducing the weight, and lessening the cholesterol levels and blood pressure. It is a fact that when cholesterol levels are high and the consumption of meat makes inflammation worse which in turn has the potential to result in pain and thus hinder the performance of every athlete as well as the time they need to recover. On the other hand, according to studies, following a diet based on plants may lead to an anti-inflammatory effect.

The thickness and viscosity of the blood are improved by following a diet based on plants, which is naturally free of cholesterol and low in saturated fat. The performance of every athlete is improved since a reduced thickness and viscosity of the blood will lead to more oxygen flowing through the muscles. Another bonus for athletes that follow a plant-based diet is the improvement of the arterial diameter and flexibility, thus improving the blood flow. According to studies, even a meal filled with fat such as egg McMuffins and sausage, it hinders for a couple of hours the arterial function.

When you compare people who base their diet on plants to people who eat meat and foods related to meat, the first group is able to get even more antioxidants. Antioxidants help in the neutralization of free radicals which lead to weakened recovery, muscle fatigue, as well as reduced athletic endurance and performance. It is also a known fact that athletes have to keep track of their weight and thus diets that are based on plants consumption will be able to help them with this task since they are high in fibers and low in fat.

This situation will lead to lessened body fat. Less body fat will translate to an increase in the aerobic capacity of the athletes and their ability to fuel their exercise by using oxygen more effectively. According to research every athlete who follows a diet based on plants is able to increase their VO2 max which is the largest amount of oxygen that they are able to use when they indulge in intense exercise, thus bettering their endurance.

Another reason for athletes and people in general for adopting a vegan lifestyle is for ethical reasons based on animal cruelty. Many people are frustrated because they do not have a say in the exploitation of animals and decide to go vegan so as to not be a part of something like that. A similar stance to the one we mentioned is the belief of many people that all sentient creatures deserve to live and it is their right to do so, thus killing them in order to eat them is not acceptable, especially when there are alternatives.

Other arguments based on ethical reasons include the belief that factory farming is inhumane as well as cruel. Also, the majority of people love animals and some of them cannot bear the thought of taking their pet for a walk and then go home to enjoy bacon butty. Similar to killing animals to obtain their meat, many vegans believe that dairy cows and chickens that lay eggs will lead a miserable and short life. For this reason, they believe the only way to stop this from happening is to exclude all animal products from their diets.

Another reason for many athletes as well as any other person to go vegan, except the various health benefits, is the positive impact this choice has on the environment. In order to maintain and feed animals in captivity, it is required a vast amount of land, a fact that is a contributing factor to deforestation. Another fact to consider that has to do with animal agriculture is that 8% of global water usage is required to be given as irrigation to feed crops.

Also, the large amounts of grain or corn that are required for animal agriculture need fertilizers as well as pesticides to grow fast and this helps in the defilement of our waterways. According to many vegans, if we only grew those plants for human usage, rather than support animals in captivity, many of the problems created would lessen or even be solved. In fact, the large numbers of animals in farms aid in the generation of waste and pollution. For example, the cows belching amounts help in expelling large numbers of methane each day (that passes)?? and animal agriculture equals 14% to 18% of greenhouse gas emissions that are caused by humans. Those numbers are at a higher level than the gas emissions from transportation.

When a vegan diet is carefully planned, since veganism requires some supplements such as vitamin B12 that is found in animal products, there are many health benefits to gain, some of which we mentioned before. An added health benefit that has been addressed by the World Health

Organization is that approximately one-third of cancers are able to be prevented by things we are able to control such as our diet. For example, by eating legumes often you may be able to lessen the risk of developing colorectal cancer by approximately 9% to 18%. Studies have also shown that consuming seven portions of vegetables and fruit each day will probably lessen the risk of death caused by cancer at 15%.

There are actually 96 studies conducted that found that there are high chances that vegans will benefit from the 15% less risk of dying from cancer since they eat more vegetables, legumes, and fruit than people who are not vegan. Soy products that are a part of the vegan diet may also offer added protection when it comes to breast cancer. In addition, the avoidance of particular animal products will most probably help in reducing the chances of developing colon, breast, and prostate cancers.

These facts may happen due to the fact that vegan diets do not include processed or smoked meat or meat that is cooked at high temperatures that is believed to enhance certain cancer types. Also, people who follow the vegan diet do not eat dairy products that, according to the results of some studies, enhance the risks of developing prostate cancer. However, there are also studies that show that dairy products may aid in the reduction of the risk of developing other cancers like colorectal cancer.

With this in mind, it is probable that the lower risk of developing cancer when following a vegan diet is not due to the exclusion of dairy products. The research that has been done until today is only observational and has been unable to pinpoint the true reason why vegans are at a lower risk of developing cancer. However, no matter the reason, following the vegan diet that is based on the daily consumption of fresh legumes, vegetables, and fruit will only benefit you more.

Did you know that eating fresh legumes, vegetables, fruit, and fibers is generally linked to considerably less risk of developing heart disease? Those things are included in a vegan diet. Several studies that are based on the observation and that compared vegetarians to vegans as well as to the population in general, concluded that vegans will most probably have a 75% less risk of developing high blood pressure. Still based on those studies and especially the study, "Beyond meatless, the health effects of vegan diets: findings from the Adventist cohorts" conducted from the Department of Nutrition, School of Public Health, Loma Linda University, CA 92350, USA, vegans will have a 42% less chance of perishing from heart disease.

Vegan diets can lead to the reduction of blood sugar levels, cholesterol, LDL, and total cholesterol levels when compared to other diets. This will help in the overall health of the heart since the blood pressure will remain on normal levels, as is the case with the blood sugar levels and cholesterol, hence reducing the chance of developing heart disease to the shocking level of 46%. Nuts and whole grain are also good for the heart, foods that are consumed regularly when following a vegan diet, especially when compared to the diet the general population follows.

Another area of your health that will benefit you from following a vegan diet is arthritis, according to the study "Whole-Foods, Plant-Based Diet

Alleviates the Symptoms of Osteoarthritis", conducted from Chelsea M. Clinton, Shanley O'Brien, and Mary R. Wendt. This study assigned randomly 40 people who suffered from arthritis and gave them two choices. The first choice was to keep following their omnivorous diet, while the second one was for them to follow a vegan diet based on whole-food and plants for the duration of 6 weeks. The participants who chose to follow a vegan diet reported that they were able to function better and that they developed higher energy levels than those who chose to not change their diet.

Two more studies, "Faecal microbial flora and disease activity in rheumatoid arthritis during a vegan diet" conducted by Peltonen R, Nenonen M, Helve T, Hänninen O, Toivanen P, Eerola E, and "Uncooked, lactobacilli-rich, vegan food and rheumatoid arthritis", conducted by Nenonen MT, Helve TA, Rauma AL, Hänninen OO, were focused on the effects of raw and rich in probiotics food (based on a vegan diet) on the symptoms developed by rheumatoid arthritis. It was reported by both studies that the people who belonged to the vegan group had improved to a greater extent their symptoms of morning stiffness, pain, and joint swelling than those who kept following an omnivorous diet.

As you can see a vegan diet that is based on whole and rich in probiotics food is able to lessen to a significant extent the symptoms of rheumatoid arthritis and osteoarthritis. These findings are important for the general population, but for athletes it is even more important since they are required to be at the peak of their health and maintain their bodies, as well as their minds, as strong as possible. Believe it or not, making this turn from an omnivorous diet to a vegan diet is not that hard, especially when you have a particular goal in mind and a reason for doing so.

Make the Transition to a Vegan Diet

Many people think that making the transition to a vegan diet and general lifestyle is an overnight achievement. While for some this could be the case, for others this leap from an omnivorous diet to a vegan one if done overnight may actually make them feel deprived and ultimately fail to follow it through. The majority of the world population is used to eating eggs, dairy, beef, chicken or pork in almost every meal of their every day lives, but this does not mean that adopting the vegan diet is an impossible task for them. Actually, making this transition should be a piece of cake by having a plan that would ultimately lead you to the goal you have set, calling yourself a true vegan and thus doing one of the most beneficial things you could do about the entire planet and yourself.

To start with, before you even start the actual transition, you should first educate yourself and learn as much as you can about the vegan diet, beliefs, and generally the vegan lifestyle. We have analyzed a great deal of all those things and throughout the course of this book, you will learn even more. You could talk with other people that have adopted the vegan lifestyle and familiarize yourself with veganism. By doing this, you will feel more prepared and filled with knowledge about your choice. For example, did you know that there are some basic types of veganism? Let us see them briefly.

First Type: Dietary Vegans

This type of vegans are also called "plant-based eaters". The term was created to refer to the people who exclude animal products from their diet, but still keep using them in other products like cosmetics and clothing.

Second Type: Whole-Food Vegans

This term applies to people who prefer to base their diet on whole foods such as whole grain, nuts, seeds, legumes, vegetables, and fruit.

Third Type: Junk-food Vegans

Some vegans include in their diet a large amount of processed vegan food such as vegan desserts including non-dairy ice cream and Oreo cookies, vegan meats, frozen dinners, and fries. This term is used to describe those types of vegans.

Fourth Type: Raw-food Vegans

This term is used to describe vegans that consume only foods that are prepared on temperatures below 48°C or foods that are raw.

Fifth Type: Low-fat, raw-food Vegans

Vegans falling in this type are also known as fruitarians since they limit in their diet foods high in fat such as coconuts, nuts, and avocados, and rely on a great extent on fruit. They consume other plants occasionally but on smaller amounts.

As we have stressed before, vegans avoid all foods that originate from animals such as:

- ✓ Chicken

- ✓ Shellfish

- ✓ Meat

- ✓ Fish

- ✓ Dairy

- ✓ Eggs

- ✓ Honey

Also, vegans avoid ingredients that are derived from animals and are used in some types of wine and beer, breakfast cereals, marshmallows, gummy candies, and gum such as:

- ✓ Gelatin

- ✓ Carmine

- ✓ Shellac

- ✓ Casein

- ✓ Isinglass

- ✓ Pepsin

- ✓ Whey

✓ Albumin

For further information, it may seem that by excluding animal products you are left with tofu and veggies alone, but this is not true. The fact of the matter is that there are many vegan alternatives for common dishes that can also be transformed easily. Some examples include:

✓ Veggie Burgers

✓ Bean Burritos

✓ Tomato Pizzas

✓ Nachos with Guacamole and Salsa

✓ Hummus Wraps

✓ Pasta Dishes

✓ Sandwiches

Entrées that are based on meat can be transformed easily with meals including:

✓ Lentils

✓ Tempeh

✓ Beans

✓ Tofu

✓ Nuts

✓ Seitan

✓ Seeds

There are many vegan choices through which you can choose such as replacing dairy products with plant milk, honey with sweeteners that are based on plants such as maple syrup or molasses, scrambled eggs with scrambled tofu, or raw eggs with chia seeds or flax.

Also, another area you should educate yourself with is knowing how to discern if a product is vegan or not by reading the ingredient lists and become familiar with understanding the less famous ingredients that are derived from animals, making an appearance on products you would not suspect them having such ingredients. For instance, a product is appropriate for vegans if it does not contain animal products and by-products or if it has not been tested on animals. All unprocessed plant food is suitable for vegan including seeds, nuts, fruit, legumes, vegetables, and beans.

Problems start when it comes to packaged food, anyway there are ways to be certain that the food you buy is appropriate for vegan consumption or not. You should start first by checking the label and packaging of the product. Since veganism has undergone a considerable boost in the number of people adopting it, the products that are labeled as vegan are increasing too. For example, you should be on the lookout for products with the label "Suitable for Vegans" or have the logo "Certified Vegan".

Another thing you should be on the lookout for is the allergen information. Products have allergy information close to the bottom of the ingredient list.

For example, if the product includes the ingredients of milk, shellfish, or eggs it will only say "Contains milk, eggs, and shellfish". An advice would be to read this first in order for you to know if you should read the ingredients list or not.

When you read the ingredients keep in mind that there are many by-products coming from animals that may confuse you at first. There is an extremely comprehensive guide on those products given by PETA Organization - People for the Ethical Treatment of Animals - and we will mention the most common ingredients you will encounter:

- ✓ Food Additives, such as E322, E542, E120, E471, E904, E631, E901, and E422.

- ✓ Carmine or Cochineal: To make carmine, which is a natural dye with the purpose of giving a red color to food products, ground cochineal scale insects are utilized.

- ✓ Gelatin: It comes from the bones, skin, and connective tissues of pigs and cows.

- ✓ Isinglass: This substance that looks like gelatin comes from the bladders of fish and is utilized often in the creation of wine and beer.

- ✓ Castoreum: This is a food flavoring that is derived from the secretions of the beavers' anal scent glands.

- ✓ Omega-3 fatty acids: The majority of the products that include Omega-3 fatty acids are not appropriate for vegans since omega-3 stems from fish. Those that are derived from algae are appropriate for vegans.

✓ Shellac: This substance is extracted by the female lac insect.

✓ Vitamin D3: Most of the D3 vitamins stem from the lanolin in sheep's wool or fish oil. There is Vitamin D3 and D2 extracted from lichen that is appropriate for vegans.

✓ There are also foods that may sometimes contain animal-derived ingredients such as:

✓ Bread products: Bread and Bagels are sometimes made including L-cysteine, which is an amino acid coming often from the feathers of poultry.

✓ Wine and Bread: Some manufacturers make wine or brew beer, using casein, egg white albumen, or gelatin. Sometimes they use isinglass but none of these products is appropriate for vegans.

✓ Caesar dressing: There are varieties of the Caesar dressing that use anchovy as an ingredient.

✓ Candy: Sometimes gummy bears, Jell-O, marshmallows, or chewing gum are made with gelatin or are coated in shellac. Sometimes carmine is used.

✓ French Fries: Often cooked in animal fat.

✓ Olive tapenade: There are many varieties that include anchovies.

- ✓ Pesto: There are varieties of pesto that may include Parmesan cheese.

- ✓ Deep-fried foods: The batter that is used to make such foods like vegetable tempura and onion rings may include eggs.

- ✓ Non-dairy creamer: There are many labeled non-dairy creamers that include casein which is a protein stemming from milk

- ✓ Pasta: Especially fresh pasta and some other types include eggs.

Another thing you should look out for is cosmetics and personal care items that should be vegan and cruelty-free. You could start making sure of that by checking the packaging and label of the product. You should look out for products that have the logo "Certified Vegan". You should not be assured if the product has a simple label of it being "vegan" or "contains no animal ingredients". You should still read the ingredient list just to be sure of it. You could even do your own research from home since PETA has also a very comprehensive list of all vegan personal care products.

When it comes to animal testing, you should search for products that are labeled with PETA's cruelty free bunny logo or with the Coalition for Consumer Information on Cosmetics (CCIC) leaping bunny logo. If the product is simply labeled as "Not tested on animals" or as "Cruelty Free", watch out because those terms are not regulated. Also, keep in mind that sometimes products not tested on animals and products that are appropriate for vegans are not necessarily exclusive since there are some cosmetics that may be cruelty free but still include some ingredients that are derived from animals. Some of the most common ingredients you should watch out for are:

- ✓ Lanolin

- ✓ Musk

- ✓ Tallow

- ✓ Keratin

- ✓ Beeswax

- ✓ Pearls

- ✓ Leather

- ✓ Silk

- ✓ Angora

- ✓ Cashmere Cashmereh

- ✓ Fur

- ✓ Wool

It would also be very beneficial for you to watch some vegan documentaries, buy some vegan magazines and books, or visit some vegan blogs, websites, and forums. They will offer you valuable information and support thus making you more confident in making this transition. Also, you should check local stores that are able to provide you with vegan products as well as research some restaurants that are vegan friendly.

After you feel you have obtained a satisfying level of knowledge on the vegan diet and lifestyle in general, it would be better to make a steady and slow transition and than cut out meat and all dairy products from your diet. In other words, you should go at a pace you feel comfortable with. If you are sure that you are able to make this change instantly without feeling deprived and fail in doing so, then, of course, feel free to act accordingly.

However, if we told most people to go to the market and not purchase dairy, meat, and eggs, then they would probably feel deprived and overwhelmed. On the other hand, if we told them to buy kale, sweet potatoes, flax, quinoa, spinach, bananas, mushrooms, coconut meat, berries, tomatoes, and almonds, they would be more confident since they would know what to shop for and what they should expect.

In most cases, it would be better to include more legumes, whole grain, seeds, nuts, tofu, and beans into your diet in order to become familiar with their uses, preparation, as well as storage. You could start by eating less meat each day and switching from milk to a non-dairy one like soy or almond milk. This is one of the first changes that feels easy to most people.At the beginning, it would be better to avoid vegan replacement meats as much as you can and replace it instead with foods that are based on plants such as vegetables, fruits, legumes, seeds, or nuts not become too addicted to them.

You could also start by being vegetarian and when you feel ready, move on being vegan by cutting off eggs and dairy one by one. For instance, you could exclude all meat from your diet along with poultry and fish. Keep in mind that you should not increase the pace you eat dairy products and eggs to replace meat. Instead, you should focus on adding more sources of protein that are based on plants. Then, you could continue with paying attention to the ingredients lists of products and avoid the ones that include rennet, gelatin, or other animal products while still keeping eggs and dairy in your diet. If you haven't done so yet, start including more beans, tofu, seeds, nuts, whole grains, and legumes in your diet. Later, start cutting off dairy products, honey, and eggs until you feel comfortable cutting them out completely. Do not forget that you should do this once you feel comfortable doing so, ideally when you feel like you do not "miss" meat and its by-products.

Making the transition from an omnivore diet to a vegan one all in once, some people find it helpful to rely on vegan hot dogs, burgers, cheeses, deli slices, or similar foods. However, keep in mind that these products are highly processed. When you are ready and comfortable with your vegan lifestyle and diet, try to lessen the use of those foods. When these products are eaten in moderation, there is nothing wrong with them, but you shouldn't get used to them being your essential source of protein, vitamins, and minerals in the long-term.

Also, you should never forget what was your motivation to begin this change. Even though losing weight is not reason enough to adopt this lifestyle since there are ways to gain weight through a vegan diet, you should keep in mind that a vegan lifestyle is almost completely different from simply starting a diet. People are generally tempted in straying from the mindset of going on a diet and cheat, but this does not apply to veganism. This is happening due to the fact that most people making the transition to veganism know the exact reason why they wish to be vegan and this way, you don't just stray from this lifestyle.

If you are still unsure of the reason, the simplest solution for you would be the first step we mentioned in this chapter: educating yourself about the various reasons people turn to veganism as we mentioned in the previous chapter and the benefits this lifestyle has on your health, humanity, and on the environment. The moment you will realize the effects that the usage of animal products has on us and on the environment, veganism will simply stick with you.

According to the British Dietetic Association, "Well-planned vegan diets can support healthy living in people of all ages". For instance, in a diet that is heavily based on animal products and thus leading to excess consumption of protein will, in turn, produce higher levels of nitrogen than the body needs. This will exhaust the kidneys which will have to get rid of the extra nitrogen with urine causing the function of the kidneys to be reduced. If this situation continues for years, people who eat high amounts of animal protein will be at a high risk of losing kidney functions permanently. Diets that are based on the consumption of high levels of animal protein will increase urine acidity. Due to the elevated acidity, the uric acid will not dissolve as easy and will turn into kidney stones.

Another thing to keep in mind is that dairy products and meat have saturated animal fats that will increase cholesterol and thus raise the risks of strokes and developing heart disease by making it difficult for the blood to flow through the arteries. If the blood is not able to flow through the heart, then the risk of a heart attack is extremely high as the same happens when the blood flow to the brain is hindered and the chances of having a stroke are extremely high too. Also, cholesterol exists only in animal products such as eggs, meat, poultry, fish, and dairy products. On the other hand, products that come from plants do not have cholesterol.

Maintaining a positive attitude throughout this whole experience is important too. Keep thinking of all the amazingly tasty foods you will be able to try and forget about the foods that you will give up. It will be a small price to pay for all the benefits you will see on your health and you will also be able to be a part of a community that is trying to save the environment and protect animals from human cruelty. Be excited about all the changes you will make and stop worrying about them. You are doing this transition for a reason and you should never forget that.

A planned transition along with remembering your goal will multiply your chances of sticking with veganism for the rest of your life. Following a vegan diet is not hard and it only becomes difficult because we make it so. Try not to overwhelm yourself and try not to rush things. Just take steady steps day by day or even better make changes, even small ones, at every meal you have. You shouldn't feel intimidated or stressed throughout the process of becoming vegan. You are changing your life in a better way and to make an impact on the world. An important thing to keep in mind is to plan your vegan diet in order to get all the necessary nutrition. This is essential for athletes that have more needs when it comes to nutrition than the average person so as to be at their peak when they train and perform.

Veganism and Sports Nutrition

It is an important fact that many professional coaches, as well as athletes, admit that nutrition in sports is essential, since food is extremely important to an athlete's overall performance, because it will provide them with the necessary energy they need, no matter which sport we deal with. Sports nutrition is different from the nutrition provided in diets that aim to increase your health in general.

The practice and study of fueling and hydrating your body with the goal of improving athletic performance is called sports nutrition and it is tasked with providing the athlete with the necessary tools to achieve his or her peak. A nutrition plan that is centered on the athlete is usually provided by an expert that is usually called "Accredited Sports Dietitian" in the sports world. Athletes have performance goals and active lifestyles that should be maintained through a balanced diet. Sports nutrition has many benefits for the athletes. Here we have some:

- ✓ It helps athletes training harder and for longer periods

- ✓ It delays the initial stages of tiredness

- ✓ It helps in the maintenance of a healthy immune system

- ✓ It improves performance

- ✓ It enhances recovery

- ✓ It improves the composition of the body

✓ It lessens the chances of a potential injury

✓ It helps with concentration and focus

Each person has different needs depending on lifestyle, age, sport, gender, and genetics among other things. For this reason, a personalized lifestyle and nutrition plan is essential, especially when the athlete follows a vegan lifestyle at early stages. For instance, recovery nutrition is extremely important for every athlete, since it refills the energy stores and nutrients that are utilized for competition or training. The best plan targeting recovery nutrition will depend on many things including the duration of the training sessions, the type of training sessions, the goals of body composition, and the time in between training sessions. The ultimate task of recovery nutrition is to fuel as well as repair the muscles and to replace the lost fluids. If the recovery nutrition plan is not the right one, it will have a negative effect on the performance of the athlete and he or she will feel tired thus affecting his or her performance.

Also, keep in mind that athletes need approximately double the amount of protein from people who are not athletes and it must be taken in the right amount and at the right time. However, the weight itself is not a determining factor to indicate how healthy an athlete is. What matters is what constitutes the athlete's weight such as having too little muscle or too much fat. Building muscle is not just a matter of protein and also includes:

✓ An added resistance to muscles

✓ Maintaining an appropriate energy balance to enhance the production of anabolic hormone

- ✓ A good distribution of nutrients in order to maintain the health of the tissues

- ✓ Enough sleep

- ✓ Having protein at the correct amounts and on the right time

There are many things athletes should watch out for, so making the transition from an omnivorous diet to a vegan one should be even better planned than the one of an average person. However, this does not indicate that the vegan diet is forbidding to athletes. Actually, there are many athletes who have adopted the vegan diet and way of life and have successfully proven that veganism is for everyone. Such an example is the famous Formula One driver Lewis Hamilton who is an avid supporter of veganism and he is dedicated to educate and encourage as many people as possible to make this transition that is beneficial for the environment and for our health.

Lewis Carl Davidson Hamilton was born in 1985 and is a British racing driver who races in Formula One for Mercedes-AMG Petronas Motorsport. He has won the Formula One World Champion six times and he is generally considered as one of the best drivers in the history of this sport of all time. He won his first title while with McLaren in 2008 and in 2013, he moved on to Mercedes. He has a tally of 151 podium finishes and 84 race victories. At the time he holds the records for the all-time most pole positions - 88, the all-time most career points - 3.431, the most points in a season - 413, and the most grand slams in a season - 3.

Despite his growing career, Lewis Hamilton made an important transition in his life when he decided to go vegan and also support veganism as publicly as he can. In 2017 during an interview, Lewis Hamilton confessed to BBC that he had decided to be vegan due to the fact that,

"I stopped eating red meat two years ago. I have generally been pescatarian for the majority of the year and now I've cut fish. As the human race, what we are doing to the world... the pollution [in terms of emissions of global-warming gases] coming from the amount of cows that are being produced is incredible.

They say it is more than what we produce with our flights and our cars, which is kind of crazy to think. The cruelty is horrible and I don't necessarily want to support that and I want to live a healthier life. So far I don't feel as if I have been missing out. But I don't know how easy it is going to be when I get home. That is going to be a real test.

Every person I have met who has gone vegan says it is the best decision they have ever made. When you watch this documentary and you see meat clogging up your arteries, you see all the stuff they put in the meat, stuff we are all eating, there is no way I am going to disregard that. I don't want in 10 or 20 years to have diabetes or catch any of that stuff.

I can continue to decide to eat that stuff and take that risk, but when you get [a disease or illness like that], you want to make a change, so I am trying to pre-empt that. I think it's the right direction and by letting people know, maybe that will encourage a couple of people to do the same thing."

The various interviews he has given where he talked about veganism as well as its benefits on the environment and to our health has inspired many people to do the same, however, words are not the only tool he uses to support veganism and what it stands for. He is opening his own vegan restaurants too. According to him, "As someone who follows a plant-based diet, I believe we need a healthier high street option that tastes amazing but also offers something exciting to those who want to be meat-free every now and again." He was working with several investors and has launched "Neat Burger". During a press release, his idea was described as the "first plant-based sustainable burger chain of its kind".

The first outlet of "Neat Burger" opened at London's Regent Street on 2 September of 2019 and it is planned to open 14 franchises all over the United States, Europe, and the Middle East for the next two years. The burgers that are included on the menu of his restaurant are produced with the collaboration of the plant-based meat alternative company "Beyond Meat". According to the words of Lewin Hamilton, "Beyond Meat is an incredible partner and I can't wait to work with the team to expand Neat Burger internationally."

Hamilton has also collaborated with the hospitality organization "The Cream Group" to launch "Neat Burger". According to Ryan Bishti, member of The Cream Group, "Neat Burger aims to change the way we view our eating habits. We're not preaching or shaming people for eating meat. We're offering an alternative that tastes as good as, if not better than meat."

Hamilton has characterized his decision to go vegan as one of the best decisions he could have made and it is second to only moving to the Mercedes team. More specifically, "I feel the best I've ever felt physically and mentally," he said in an interview. "All year I've felt very strong mentally, but I think physically I'm now taking also a big step and that's really the decision I made to change my diet."

The example Lewis Hamilton provides us with is an admirable one as well as the example many other athletes and celebrities from all over the world. However, there is still doubt whether veganism is able to support the higher needs of athletes when compared to other people or not. For instance, some coaches doubt the fact that athletes are able to get all the necessary amounts of macronutrients - protein, fat, and carbohydrate - from a vegan diet and the same applies to the micronutrients - vitamins, phytonutrients, minerals, etc.

We will prove that there should be no doubt and with the right amount of planning and caution, as is the case for omnivorous diets too, athletes will be able to get the necessary and right amount of nutrition to be at their best health and performance. However, keep in mind that nowadays there is little evidence if at all to prove that the various types of vegetarian and vegan diets are better than the various types of the omnivorous diets. So, what we are trying to accomplish is proving that the vegan diet can be and already is as nutritious as the omnivorous diet, especially for athletes that have much more demands on this matter than people who are not athletes.

Some general guidelines that we will analyze in more detail later include that all athletes, no matter their level, age, and status, are able to meet their nutrient and energy needs while following a vegan diet that includes a wide variety of foods such as vegetables, fruits, and plant foods that are rich in protein.

For athletes that require high levels of energy for their respective sport, they may need to eat meals frequently as well as consume snacks and lessen the amounts of foods that are rich in fiber. Also, some particular nutrients such as omega-3 fatty acids, vitamin D, protein, iodine, riboflavin, zinc, iron, calcium, and vitamin B12, when compared to animal foods, they are found less in plants or they are absorbed less well. Normally, a vegan diet that is well planned and includes foods that contain those nutrients will provide an athlete with the necessary amounts. However, an added supplement of those nutrients may be needed occasionally.

Various short-term intervention and observational studies that have been conducted on athletes that have followed vegetarian and omnivorous diets for a test period of several weeks have concluded that there is no difference in the power, anaerobic, strength, and aerobic performance of those people based on whether their diet includes or excludes meat and its by-products. It has been hypothesized by observation and research that the various vegetarian diets, including, the vegan diet, are able to help athletes to improve their performance and training because of the high content of antioxidants, carbohydrates, and other phytochemicals, not to mention the alkaline earth metal strontium.

An ergogenic advantage that can be attributed to vegetarian diets is the inclusion of a serum, small in amount, alkalinity at the duration of the exercise of athletes. When compared to an omnivorous diet, the antioxidants in a plant-based diet are higher and this may help in lessening the oxidative stress that is often attributed to intense and long exercise as well as regulate inflammation and immune function. However, keep in mind that a diet based on plants may impair the performance and health of the athlete if the foods that are included in the diet are not appropriate and less optimal for his or her needs.

All athletes make their priority to meet the necessary energy needs when it comes to nutrition. When athletes do not take the necessary energy for them, the benefits of training are nullified, their performance is affected and even worse, their health could be affected by the loss of bone density or muscle mass. They are also at risk of illness, fatigue, and injury. The energy levels athletes need to have daily, are different among each one and they also depend on the sport each athlete is dedicated to. Another factor of the energy levels is the intensity of training as well as how often their training takes place, which will likely vary from season to season. Other general factors that have to do with the required energy are body composition, age, and sex.

It is true that some vegan athletes that need high energy levels may not be able to meet those energy needs because of the low energy and high fiber density of diets based on plants, but this shouldn't be forbidding to athletes that require high energy levels. They should deal with this setback by eating snacks and meals frequently, such as 5 to 8 meals and snacks each day, and plan their food as well as snacks beforehand so as for them to be ready and available to he athletes whenever they are needed. For example, an athlete can pack small meals and snacks in his or her backpack or gym bag and have them ready to provide the necessary food energy.

Also, limiting the foods that are rich in fiber and selecting foods dense with energy may also help in meeting the required energy levels. For instance, the athlete can replace with fruit juice several whole fruit portions and eat one-third to one-half of breads, grains, and cereals. It could also help to consume less processed sources like sourdough bread or white rice than brown rice and whole wheat bread since it will lessen the intake of excessive fiver as well as the early signs of satiety.

On the other hand, other vegan athletes may need less energy to maintain a slow reduction of their weight for health or training reasons. In such cases, the athletes will benefit more from concentrating more on including foods that are unprocessed and whole in order to achieve healthy body weight and incite satiety. An example of a 3,000 Kcal meal day for athletes following the vegan diet is the following one:

<u>Breakfast</u>

The athlete will need:

- ✓ 57 grams of Grains

- ✓ 57 grams of Proteins

- ✓ ½ cups of Vegetables

- ✓ 1 cup of Fruit

- ✓ ½ cup of Dairy Equipment

This translates to:

- ✓ 2 slices of whole-wheat toast with margarine and 1 spoonful of fruit preserves

- ✓ ½ cup of scrambled tofu

- ✓ ½ cup of peppers and spinach

- ✓ 1 cup of orange juice that is fortified with calcium

- ✓ Latte which is created with ½ cup of soymilk

<u>Lunch</u>:

The athlete will need:

- ✓ 57 grams of Grains

- ✓ 57grams of Proteins

- ✓ 1 cup of Vegetables

- ✓ 1 cup of Fruit

- ✓ ½ cup of Dairy Equipment

This translates to:

✓ 2 slices of sourdough bread

✓ 2 cups of Minestrone Soup which is created with 1/h cup of garbanzo beans, ¼ cup of kidney beans, ¾ cup of various vegetables and olive oil.

✓ Large apple

<u>Snack</u>:

The athlete will need:

✓ 57 grams of Grains

✓ 29 grams of Proteins

✓ ½ cup of Dairy Equipment

This translates to:

✓ 57 grams of a large whole-grain bagel

✓ 1 spoonful of peanut butter

✓ 1 cup of soymilk

<u>Dinner</u>:

The athlete will need:

91

✓ 114 grams of Grains

✓ 57 grams of Protein

✓ 2 and half cups of Vegetables

This translates to:

4 Lentil Tacos which are cooked with:

✓ Tomato sauce,

✓ Onion celery,

✓ Lentils,

✓ Canned tomatoes,

✓ Canola oil on corn tortillas

They are served with:

✓ Fresh tomato,

✓ Salsa,

✓ Jicama,

✓ Avocado,

✓ Lettuce

<u>Snack</u>:

The athlete will need:

- ✓ 1 cup of Dairy Equipment

This translates to:

- ✓ 1 cup of Rice Yogurt

- ✓ ½ cup of sliced peaches or berries

<u>Snacks that have to do with exercise</u>:

- ✓ Sports gels

- ✓ Beverage of fluid replacement

- ✓ Sports bars

This is a sample meal plan for Vegans using United States Department of Agriculture "MyPlate" and before following any meal plan you should consult an expert because for each athlete a meal plan is unique and should be created according to the various other factors we mentioned and are included for creating the ideal personalized diet for each athlete and his or her respective sport.

Another important part of the diet athletes should follow are carbohydrates and they should be the largest component of their energy intake. Thus, the ingestion of carbohydrates is extremely important for an athlete to achieve optimal performance when he or she is engaged to high-intensity or moderate exercise that takes more than 90 minutes to complete as well as during intermittent activities that are high in intensity which is usually the case for various team sports. Another part carbohydrates are essential for is the refilling of glycogen after exercising and also they are able to make sure the athlete has adapted adequately to his or her training.

There are several factors that determine the amount of carbohydrates athletes should have on their daily meals and some of them include the kind of sport they are engaged to, the intensity of their training, and their body mass (BM). Currently, the recommendation of carbohydrates for athletes that perform moderate to high-intensity training of 1 to 3 hours each day is 5 to 10 grams of carbohydrate/kg BM/day. Fewer amounts of 3 to 5 grams per kg BM are recommended for athletes that perform low-intensity training or one that is based on skills. Higher amounts of carbohydrates of 8 to 12 grams per kg BM are appropriate for athletes that undergo extreme endurance training.

Even though the vegan diet is filled with carbohydrates, it is very important to make sure that you are ingesting enough carbohydrates due to the rise of diets that are low on carbohydrates and can also seem appealing to several vegan athletes. For this reason, it is extremely important on consulting an expert for every change you wish to make on your diet so as to ensure that your intake of carbohydrates is the appropriate one.

The requirements each athlete has when it comes to protein are different and based on his or her type of activity and training level. Generally, an athlete that goes through intense hours of training will require more protein when compared to a person that is engaging in moderate exercises for some days each week. For people who exercise for several times each week with a light to moderate intensity, the United States Recommended Dietary Allowance (RDA) recommend an intake of 0.8 g protein/kg BM/day. On the other hand, athletes that train at a higher intensity will need more protein than the group of people we mentioned before. Studies based on the intake of protein athletes should acquire, have shown that protein interacts with exercise and provide them with an exceptional base for the synthesizing of contractile, metabolic and structural proteins. Protein is also essential for triggering the protein synthesis of muscles.

At the time, the recommendations for protein intake by athletes include 1.2-2.0 g protein/kg BM/day. These recommendations are appropriate for the support of the metabolic repair, remodeling, adaptation as well as protein turnover. There is little to no evidence that shows the recommended protein intake for athletes that follow the vegan diet should be any different from the athletes who follow an omnivorous diet also taking into consideration the wide range of protein sources that are suggested to athletes. in order to make sure that athletes take the necessary amount of protein suited for their needs, they should consume a wide range of foods that are plant-based and rich in protein throughout the day. Athletes should be encouraged to make combinations such as beans with seeds or nuts or make a peanut butter sandwich.

Another important nutrition part for athletes is the fat intake that should be similar to the one recommended to the public health guidelines. Fat intake is personalized for each athlete and depends on the goal of body composition and training. Fat is essential since it is able to provide many elements of cell membranes, energy, and essential fatty acids as well as it helps in the absorption of vitamins that are fat-soluble.

The fat that is stored in adipocytes and active muscle works as a source of energy throughout long exercises of low-level activities and moderate in intensity ones. Out of the total energy intake, according to the U.S. Department of Health and Human Services and the U.S. Department of Agriculture, less than 10% should be saturated fat and emphasis should be given to essential fatty acids in our diet in order to meet the general recommendations. Even though very low in fat, vegan diets are recommended in order to treat and prevent diabetes and cardiovascular disease, should be avoided by athletes since they are very restrictive, especially for those that undergo intense training routines.

Vegan athletes are certain to obtain the necessary fat intake through a wide range of source selection that is based on plants. However, the vegan diet may be rich in omega-6 polyunsaturated fatty acids, but it lacks in omega-3 fatty acids, which are important for inflammatory modulation. Also, vegan athletes should consider supplements of DHA-rich microalgae that are able to be absorbed well and increase the concentrations of eicosapentaenoic acid (EPA) and docosahexaenoic acid (DHA) in the blood.

As we have discussed minerals and vitamins are also essential on a balanced diet and this does not exclude athletes under any circumstances.

Iron intake is essential, especially for female vegan athletes. The iron that is based on plants or else non-heme iron could be easily absorbed with the consumption of foods containing ascorbic acids such as tomatoes, melon, juice, or citrus fruit, as well as other organic acids. It can be hindered by the following:

- ✓ Plant phytates

- ✓ Tannins in tea

- ✓ Polyphenolics

- ✓ Cocoa

- ✓ Coffee

- ✓ Dairy protein

- ✓ Soy

It can also be obstructed by foods that have a high concentration of zinc and calcium as well as other divalent minerals. If you are able to cook with iron cookware it will help you to enhance the iron content, especially with foods that are acidic such as tomato sauce. If you think that iron is something you should be concerned about, a sports physician or dietitian will be able to assess if an athlete needs additional supplementation. You should not take the liberty to take iron supplements on your own unless you are diagnosed with iron deficiency since it will probably get in the way of the absorption of other minerals.

Zink is also essential to athletes and as is the case with iron, zinc intake may be lacking in certain athletes, especially female ones and those who follow vegan diets. In the case of vegan athletes, a deficiency in zinc intake may be a result of reduced availability of zinc by plants when they are compared to animal foods or including to their diet foods that have little to no zinc.

Vegan athletes who follow a balanced and varied sourced diet that includes a wide range of plant foods that are rich in zinc such as whole grains and legumes have higher chances of reaching the appropriate zinc intake without needing added supplementation. Organic acids like lactic, citric, and malic acids will be able to improve the absorption of zinc to a certain level, as it happens with iron too. Keep in mind that some techniques of food preparation like the sprouting and soaking of beans, nuts, seeds, and grains or the leavening of bread will hinder the binding of zinc by phytic acid.

One of the most common concerns for vegan athletes is the intake of calcium since they consume no dairy products. It is possible for vegans to get the necessary calcium intake they require through a wise selection of sources of calcium that are absorbed well enough combined with the use of foods that are calcium-fortified such as fortified orange juice with calcium citrate malate, nuts, or fortified soymilk. Rich in calcium plant foods can be as good as or sometimes better than cows milk which has an absorption rate of 32% with the exception of beet greens, spinach, rhubarb, and chard that have a low bioavailability of less than 5% to 8% because of the high amounts of oxalate content.

Vitamin D is also important since it helps in the absorption of calcium and can also pose a concern of some athletes because of the limited exposure to the sun or the fewer consumption of foods that contain Vitamin D. Even though vegan athletes may be at a higher risk of not acquiring the necessary Vitamin D intake due to dietary reasons, there are other factors to consider such as sun exposure ratio, skin pigmentation, and dietary supplementation which are more essential to the level of vitamin D than its intake form several food sources. You will be able to obtain the necessary vitamin D for you through exposing your back, abdomen, arms, and legs to the sunlight for approximately 10 to 30 minutes several times each week by wearing shorts and a sports bra, always depending on skin pigmentation.

For athletes who use sunscreen in high amounts, live at high altitudes, train for the most part indoors, have fair skin or a dark pigmented one, have photosensitivity, or have excess body fat, supplementation may be needed. Vegan athletes can also seek vitamin D-3 better from lichen that lanolin and D-2 from irradiation of yeast ergosterol. However, according to research vitamin D-2 can be less effective when ingested in higher doses than vitamin D-3.

An insufficient iodine level can be commonly observed in vegan athletes who do not eat table salt that is fortified with iodine, consume plant foods that have been cultivated in soil with poor iodine amounts or do not consume sea vegetables. As evidence suggests, iodine can be lost with sweat thus placing athletes who sweat too much at an even greater risk for having low levels of iodine. Athletes will be able to make sure they receive the appropriate amount of iodine for them by using iodized salt when cooking. For instance, ½ spoonful or 3 grams will provide 1,180 mg of sodium. They could also lessen the consumption of processed foods. Gourmet salts, salty seasonings such as soy sauce and tamari, and sea salt, as well as processed foods that contain sodium, are not iodized.

The most common deficiency amongst vegan athletes is the vitamin B-12 one since this vitamin is found only in animal products. For this reason, athletes should be encouraged to consume foods that are fortified with vitamin B-12, take a supplement containing vitamin B-12, or take a multivitamin. Riboflavin should also be considered by vegan athletes since they do not consume dairy products. Keep in mind that the riboflavin can be found in small amounts in most plant foods and for this reason an expert will plan your diet accordingly.

Vegan athletes will be able to reach the necessary nutrient and energy intake with careful planning. For this reason, athletes should follow a diet that includes a wide range of plant foods and enriched grain products along with vegetables, fruits, and plant foods that are rich in proteins. Trainers and professionals should be able to understand and be sensitive to the reasons why an athlete has chosen to become a vegan, as well as educate vegan athletes of the various sources of micronutrients and macronutrients.

This is why athletes should not worry about not getting enough support from their coaches and let this be a reason for not making this important transition that will benefit themselves and the environment. This choice rests with the athletes and is a personal one. Meeting energy requirements is a crucial step to gain optimal performance and acquire proper nutrition. This is why trainers should be informed of the different sources and choices an athlete has when he or she decides to make a change in his or her diet.

Sources of Nutrition in the Vegan Diet

The key factor for a vegan diet to be able to meet the nutrient goals of nearly any person no matter his or her age is a well-planned and balanced vegan diet. The truth of the matter is that despite any misconceptions people have, a healthy and balanced vegan diet is able to provide all the needed energy for the average person as well as for athletes.

Some of the most common questions that have to do with veganism include, "How are vegans able to get B12?", "How are vegans able to get protein?", "How are vegans able to get calcium since they have excluded milk from their diets?". All vegans need to meet their nutritional requirements. They need a diet full of legumes, fruits, nuts, a number of fortified foods, vegetables, seeds, and complex carbohydrates or a multi-vitamin.

We will present a list of various foods that will be able to provide vegans with the different necessary nutrients and should be included in various vegan diets according to experts. However, do not attempt to make your own meal plan because, especially athletes, should consult an expert that will take into consideration more than just the number of proteins fats or carbohydrates a food has.

To start with, nearly all foods include at least small amounts of protein. Foods such as beans, nuts, soy, seeds, grains, and legumes are all amazing sources of protein. Take, for example, a banana sandwich that is made from 2 slices of whole-grain bread and peanut butter, has 18 grams to 22 grams of protein. The thing you will need to keep in mind is that basing your diet to a variety of foods that are based on plants, you will be able to reach or even exceed the recommended protein intakes.

For instance, for a person who follows a diet based on plants, it is advisable to have an intake of 0.9 grams per kilogram of body weight. However, this applies to an average person and athletes who are extremely active will most probably have to intake more protein in order to be able and support their activity level, so an expert will be able to pinpoint exactly the amount of protein they will need. Below is a list of the various foods that can be used as a protein source in a vegan diet:

Seitan:

It is very popular among many vegans as well as vegetarians. Seitan is created from gluten which is the essential protein in wheat. Seitan can be compared to the texture and look of meat when it is cooked unlike other mock meats that are based in soy. Other names for seitan include wheat gluten or wheat meat and it has 25 grams of protein per 100 grams.

This fact makes it a food that is extremely rich in protein. This alternative meat can also be an adequate source of selenium and contains small proportions of calcium, iron, and phosphorus. Seitan can be sautéed, fried on a pan, and grilled, thus making it an easy addition to many recipes. However, people who are sensitive to gluten or have celiac disease should avoid seitan.

Edamame, Tofu, and Tempeh:

Edamame, Tofu, and Tempeh originate from soybeans. Soybeans are able to provide us with all the essential amino acids the body needs since they are considered to be a whole source of protein. Edamame are the immature soybeans and have a delicately sweet and grassy taste. Before eating them, they should be boiled or steamed and can make a fine addition to salads or be consumed on their own.

With a production process that resembles cheese making, tofu is created by bean curds that are pressed together. Tempeh is created by cooking and lightly fermenting the mature soybeans before they are pressed in a patty. Tempeh's flavor resembles one of the nuts while tofu doesn't have a particular taste, but is able to absorb the flavor of the various ingredients that are prepared with it. Tempeh and tofu can be a fine addition to many recipes, from chilies and burgers to soups.

All three include calcium, iron and 10 grams to 19 grams of protein per 100 grams. Also, edamame are particularly rich in vitamin K, folate, and fiber. Tempeh has a substantial amount of B vitamins, probiotics, and minerals such as phosphorus and magnesium.

Lentils:

Lentils are an amazing source of protein since each cooked cup of 240 ml has 18 grams of protein. They can make a great addition to many dishes, from dahls infused with spice, fresh salads, to soups. Another thing lentils contain is a considerable amount of carbs that are slowly digested and one cup of 240 ml will be able to provide you with about 50% of the fiber daily intake that is recommended for you.

According to research, lentils include a type of fiber that is known for providing food to the good bacteria in the colon, thus maintaining a healthy gut. Also, lentils may be able to reduce the risks of you developing, excess body weight, heart disease, certain types of cancer, and diabetes. Added to this, lentils are also rich in iron, folate, and manganese as well as they have a substantial amount of antioxidants and other plant compounds that help in the maintenance of your health.

Most Varieties of Beans and Chickpeas:

Varieties such as black, kidney, pinto, and many other beans have high amounts of protein for each serving. Otherwise known as garbanzo beans, chickpeas have content that is rich in protein as is the case with various other legumes. For each cooked cup of 240 ml, chickpeas and beans have approximately 15 grams of protein and can be also great sources of iron, complex carbs, phosphorus, fiber, manganese, folate, and potassium, among several other plant compounds that are beneficial for our health.

Several studies have indicated that when people follow a diet that is rich in beans as well as other legumes too, they have high chances of limiting cholesterol, controlling their blood sugar levels, reduce belly fat, and lower the blood pressure. You could effectively add bean into your diet by cooking a bowl of homemade chili or for extra benefits to your health add a bit of turmeric on roasted chickpeas.

Nutritional Yeast:

As nutritional yeast, we define the deactivated strain of Saccharomyces cerevisiae yeast that is sold for commercial use in the form of flakes or powder. Its taste is similar to the one of cheese, a fact that makes it quite popular as an ingredient for cooking foods such as scrambled tofu or mashed potatoes. You could also sprinkle nutritional yeast on top of pasta or use it as a topping for popcorn. The amount of protein nutritional yeast provides us with is 14 grams of protein for every 28 grams as well as 7 grams of fiber in the same amount. Fortified nutritional yeast can be an amazing source for magnesium, manganese, zinc, copper, and all the B vitamins along with B12.

Teff and Spelt:

Teff and spelt belong to a group of grains that is called as ancient grains. Some other ancient grains include barley, spelt, einkorn, and sorghum. Spelt is a form of wheat that includes gluten, while teff comes from an annual grass and thus has no gluten in it. For each cooked cup of 240 ml teff and spelt provide us with 10 to 11 grams of protein and this makes them the highest in protein amongst the other ancient grains.

They are also great sources of other nutrients such as iron, manganese, magnesium, fiber, complex carbs, and phosphorus. In these two we could also have substantial amounts of zinc, selenium, and B vitamins. Teff and spelt can be used as alternatives to the usual grains like rice and wheat and can make a great addition to various dishes such as risotto, polenta, and other baked foods.

Hempseed:

Hempseed originates from the plant of Cannabis sativa, which is famous for belonging in the same plant family as marijuana. However, when compared to marijuana hempseed only contains some small amounts of THC, which is the compound responsible for the drug-like effects of marijuana. Despite the fact that hempseed is not as famous as other seeds it has 10 grams of easily absorbed and complete protein for every 28 grams. This amount equals to 50% more protein than flaxseeds and chia seeds.

Hempseed also has considerable amounts of calcium, magnesium, selenium, iron, and zinc. Added to this, it could be a good source of omega-6 and omega-3 fatty acids in the ratio that is considered good for our health. According to some studies that have been conducted such as

"Gamma-linolenic acid inhibits inflammatory responses by regulating NF-kappaB and AP-1 activation in lipopolysaccharide-induced RAW 264.7 macrophages," by Chang CS, Sun HL, Lii CK, Chen HW, Chen PY, Liu KL.

"Efficacy of dietary hempseed oil in patients with atopic dermatitis" by Callaway J, Schwab U, Harvima I, Halonen P, Mykkänen O, Hyvönen P, Järvinen T.

"Essential fatty acids for premenstrual syndrome and their effect on prolactin and total cholesterol levels: a randomized, double blind, placebo-controlled study" by Rocha Filho EA, Lima JC, Pinho Neto JS, Montarroyos U.

"The effects of Cannabis sativa L. seed (hempseed) in the ovariectomized rat model of menopause" by Saberivand A, Karimi I, Becker LA, Moghaddam A, Azizi-Mahmoodjigh S, Yousefi M, Zavareh S.

The types of fats that are found in hempseed will most probably be able to lessen inflammation, particular diseases of the skin, and reduce the symptoms of menopause and PMS. Hempseed can be added to your diet in various homemade salad dressings, protein bars, into your smoothie, and morning muesli.

Green Peas:

Green peas that are most commonly served as a side dish, actually have 9 grams of protein for each cooked cup of 240 ml. This amount of protein is a bit more than that of a cup of milk. Another amazing fact about the little green peas is that a serving of those will cover approximately 25% and more of your daily requirements of manganese, vitamin A - C - K, folate, fiber, and thiamine. They can also be an appropriate source of zinc, magnesium, copper, iron, phosphorus, and other B vitamins. With green peas, you could make basil and pea stuffed ravioli, avocado and pea guacamole, or a bowl of pea soup.

Spirulina:

Spirulina is an algae of blue and green color and is definitely a nutritional bomb. For instance, 30 ml or else two spoonfuls of spirulina will offer you 8 grams of complete protein and will cover your daily intake of thiamin and iron at a 22% as well as your daily needs of copper at a 42%. Spirulina also includes considerable amounts of riboflavin, potassium, magnesium, and manganese, as well as smaller amounts of most of the various other nutrients your body needs such as essential fatty acids.

In spirulina, we can find a natural pigment called phycocyanin, which seems to have strong antioxidant, anti-cancer, and anti-inflammatory properties. There are various studies that indicate the fact that spirulina offers many health benefits such as less blood pressure, a strong immune system, and improved cholesterol and blood sugar levels. Those studies include:

"The effects of Spirulina on anemia and immune function in senior citizens," by Carlo Selmi, Patrick SC Leung, [...], and M Eric Gershwin.

"Antihyperlipemic and antihypertensive effects of Spirulina maxima in an open sample of mexican population: a preliminary report" by Patricia V Torres-Duran, Aldo Ferreira-Hermosillo, and Marco A Juarez-Oropeza.

"Role of Spirulina in the Control of Glycemia and Lipidemia in Type 2 Diabetes Mellitus," by Parikh P, Mani U, Iyer U.

"The hypolipidaemic effects of Spirulina (Arthrospira platensis) supplementation in a Cretan population: a prospective study," by Mazokopakis EE, Starakis IK, Papadomanolaki MG, Mavroeidi NG, Ganotakis ES.

Quinoa and Amaranth:

Quinoa and Amaranth are often considered as free of gluten grains or ancient grains, however, they do not grow in grasses like other cereal grains. This is the reason why they are considered technically as "pseudocereals". Despite this fact, they can both be grounded into flours as many common grains we know. Quinoa and amaranth are complete sources of protein, something that can be considered as rare between pseudocereals and grains, and can provide you with 8 to 9 grams of protein for each cooked cup of 240 ml. Both quinoa and amaranth can be considered as good sources of iron, magnesium, fiber, complex carbs, manganese, as well as phosphorus.

Ezekiel Bread and Breads Created From Sprouted Grains:

Ezekiel bread is produced by sprouted and organic whole grains as well as legumes including millet, spelt, soybeans, lentils, wheat, and barley. By consuming two slices of Ezekiel bread, you will obtain 8 grams of protein, an amount that is slightly elevated when compared to an average bread.

Legumes and sprouting grains are able to increase the number of healthy nutrients they have and lessen the number of anti-nutrients as well, according to the following studies:

"New functional legume foods by germination: effect on the nutritive value of beans, lentils, and pea," by Concepción Vidal-Valverde, Juana Frias, Isabel Sierra, Inmaculada Blazquez, Fernand Lambein, and Yu-Haey Kuo.

"The presence and inactivation of trypsin inhibitors, tannins, lectins and amylase inhibitors in legume seeds during germination. A review." by Savelkoul FH1, van der Poel AF, Tamminga S.

Also, according to the study, "Changes in the carbohydrates and nitrogenous components during germination of proso millet, Panicum miliaceum." by KP1, Sadasivam S., sprouting increases their content of amino acids. Keep in mind, that lysine is the limiting amino acid that can be found in many plants and is known that sprouting can increase the content of lysine, thus boosting the quality of protein overall.

Also, by combining legumes with grains you could improve further the amino acids in bread. Another thing that sprouting is known for is the increase of the bread's vitamin C, beta-carotene, soluble fiber, vitamin E, and folate content as well as lesen slightly the content of gluten, thus enhancing digestion to the people that have problems with gluten.

Soy Milk:

An amazing alternative for cow's milk is the milk created by soybeans and is fortified with minerals and vitamins, otherwise known as soy milk. This milk offers you 7 grams of protein for each cup of 240 ml and is a great source for vitamin B12, vitamin D, and calcium. However, you should keep in mind that soybeans and soy milk do not have naturally the vitamin B12, so it would be recommended for you to pick a fortified variety. You will be able to find soy milk to most supermarkets and it is a product that can be used for baking and cooking recipes as well as consumed on its own. Also, it would be good to choose varieties without added sugars to keep their intake amount to a minimum.

Oatmeal and Oats:

Oats are a delicious way for you to add the necessary protein to your diet. For instance, 120 ml or half a cup of dry oats will provide you with about 6 grams of protein as well as 4 grams of fiber. This amount of oats will also offer you substantial amounts of folate, zinc, magnesium, and phosphorus. Even though oats are not believed to be a complete protein, they have the benefit of including protein of higher quality than other grains that are commonly consumed such as wheat and rice. Oats can be used to many recipes such as veggie burgers and oatmeal. You could also ground them into flour and use them for baking.

Wild Rice:

Wild rice is rich in protein when compared to other rice varieties such as basmati and brown rice since it has 1.5 times more protein. For instance, 240 ml or one cooked cup will give you 7 grams of protein a well as an adequate addition of manganese, phosphorus, B vitamins, fiber, magnesium, and copper. Wild rice has not its bran removed as is the case with white rice, which from a nutritional point of view is amazing since bran has many vitamins, minerals, and fiber.

However, this fact may raise some concerns that have to do with arsenic. This is happening because the bran of the rice crops that are growing in polluted areas, may gather arsenic. Arsenic may elevate the chances of developing various health problems when it is regularly consumed and for long periods of time since it is a toxic trace element according to many studies including:

"Arsenic in the aetiology of cancer," by Tapio S, Grosche B.

"Arsenic exposure and cardiovascular disorders: an overview," by Balakumar P1, Kaur J.

"Arsenic and diabetes and hypertension in human populations: a review," by Chen CJ, Wang SL, Chiou JM, Tseng CH, Chiou HY, Hsueh YM, Chen SY, Wu MM, Lai MS.

For these reasons, it would be wise to wash wild rice before cooking it and to use much more water than normal since those precautions may lessen the arsenic amounts up to 57% according to the study, "Arsenic burden of cooked rice: Traditional and modern methods," by Sengupta MK, Hossain MA, Mukherjee A, Ahamed S, Das B, Nayak B, Pal A, Chakraborti D.

Chia Seeds:

Chia seeds come from Guatemala and Mexico since the plant they come from, Salvia hispanica, is native there. Chia seeds are rich in protein since they contain 13 grams of fiber and 6 grams of protein per 35 grams. They also contain an adequate amount of calcium, magnesium, omega-3 fatty acids, selenium, iron, antioxidants, and many other plant compounds that are beneficial for our health. They can also be added in several recipes since they can absorb water pretty well and turn into a substance that resembles gel. For example, they can be added to baked foods, smoothies, or create chia puddings.

Nut Butter, Nuts, Other Seeds:

Seeds, nuts as well as the products that come from them can be great sources of protein. For instance, 28 grams of nuts contain approximately 5 to 7 grams of protein, always depending on the seed variety and the nut. Seeds and nuts can also be great sources of healthy fats, calcium, selenium, fiber, vitamin E, phosphorus, iron, magnesium, and particular B vitamins.

Amongst other plant compounds that are beneficial for our health, they contain antioxidants. Keep in mind that when you are thinking of which nuts and seeds to choose and buy, roasting and blanching have probably damaged the nutrients that nuts contain. So it would be wise to opt for unblanched and raw nuts and seeds whenever you are able to. Also, it would be wise to choose natural nut butter since you will avoid this way the excess sugar, oil, and salt that are added by many brands.

Vegetables and Fruits rich in Protein:

It is a fact that all vegetables and fruits have protein but in relatively small amounts. However, there are some that have more protein when compared to others. The vegetables that include the most protein are spinach, potatoes, broccoli, asparagus, sweet potatoes, Brussels sprouts, and artichokes. For each cooked cup, they have approximately 4 to 5 grams of protein.

Even though corn is considered a grain, sweet corn is one of the most common foods that has about the same protein levels as the vegetables we mentioned that are high in protein. Generally, fresh fruits have a lower content of protein when compared to vegetables. Fruits that have the most protein in comparison are cherimoyas, nectarines, guava, blackberries, bananas, and mulberries. All of these have approximately 2 to 4 grams of protein for each cup.

Those are the foods that can be an excellent protein source for every athlete and average person alike. In some of them, we mentioned the term "complete protein". Complete proteins have the right amount of all the 9 essential amino acids that are required for the dietary needs of humans. Nearly all the foods that are based on plants include all 9 essential amino acids, however, their proportions are different and for this reason, they are believed to be incomplete.

Keep in mind that our bodies are able to combine incomplete proteins when they are consumed within 24 hours from each other. However, you do not have to eat them this way on purpose. If you consume any plant food with the exception of fruit, you will be provided with enough of the 9 essential amino acids to achieve the necessary requirements with the condition of meeting the needed calories. As long as you are provided with enough energy, in other words calories, it will be nearly impossible to develop a deficiency in the essential amino acids.

Moving on, iron is found rich in dried beans as well as in dark green leafy vegetables and those are even considered to be even better than meat on a per calorie standpoint. The absorption of iron is increased considerably when consuming along with foods that include vitamin C. One thing that you should keep in mind from the start about iron, is that vegans are not at a higher risk than people who eat meat to develop iron deficiency. Iron can be found in two forms, non-heme iron, and heme iron.

Heme iron takes up to 40% of the iron in fish, meat, and poultry is absorbed well by our bodies. Non-heme iron that is found in plants is not as well absorbed by our bodies. Since vegan diets are based on the consumption of foods that contain only non-heme iron, vegans should consume foods high in iron and methods that can promote the absorption of iron such as consuming foods that contain also vitamin C. The iron recommendation for vegans is almost 1.8 times higher than the iron recommendation for people who are not vegans. However, vegans and particularly athletes should not be worried because the vegan diet is rich in vitamin C, which increases the absorption ratio of non-heme iron six fold. Many vegetables are high in both iron and vitamin C such as bok choy and broccoli. Below, we will provide a list of the foods that are rich as well as their content in iron measured in mg.

- ✓ Blackstrap molasses - 2 spoonful - 7.2 mg

- ✓ Tofu - ½ cup - 6.6 mg

- ✓ Cooked lentils - 1 cup - 6.6 mg

- ✓ Cooked spinach - 1 cup - 6.4 mg

- ✓ Cooked kidney beans - 1 cup - 5.2 mg

- ✓ Cooked chickpeas - 1 cup - 4.7 mg

- ✓ Cooked Soybeans - 1 cup - 4.5 mg

- ✓ Tempeh - 1 cup - 4.5 mg

- ✓ Cooked Lima beans - 1 cup - 4.5 mg

- ✓ Cooked black-eyed peas - 1 cup - 4.3 mg

- ✓ Cooked Swiss chard - 1 cup - 4.0 mg

- ✓ Enriched bagel - 1 medium - 3.8 mg

- ✓ Cooked black beans - 1 cup - 3.6 mg

- ✓ Cooked pinto beans - 1 cup - 3.6 mg

- ✓ One veggie hot dog fortified with iron - 3.6 mg

- ✓ Prune juice - 250 ml - 3.0 mg

- ✓ Cooked quinoa - 1 cup - 2.8 mg

- ✓ Cooked beet greens - 1 cup - 2.7 mg

- ✓ Tahini - 2 spoonful - 2.7 mg

- ✓ Cooked peas - 1 cup - 2.5 mg

- ✓ Cashews - 1/4 cup - 2.0 mg

- ✓ Cooked Brussels sprouts - 1 cup - 1.9 mg

- ✓ Potato with skin - 1 large - 1.9 mg

- ✓ Cooked bok choy - 1 cup - 1.8 mg

- ✓ Cooked bulgur - 1 cup - 1.7 mg

- ✓ Raisins - 1/2 cup - 1.5 mg

- ✓ Dried apricots - 15 halves - 1.4 mg

- ✓ Soy yogurt - 178 ml - 1.4 mg

- ✓ Veggie burger - 1 patty - 1.4 mg

- ✓ Watermelon - medium - 1.4 mg

- ✓ Almonds - 1/4 cup - 1.3 mg

- ✓ Sesame seeds - 2 spoonful - 1.2 mg

- ✓ Sunflower seeds - 1/4 cup - 1.2 mg

- ✓ Cooked turnip greens - 1 cup - 1.2 mg

- ✓ Cooked millet - 1 cup - 1.1 mg

- ✓ Cooked broccoli - 1 cup - 1.0 mg

- ✓ Cooked kale - 1 cup - 1.0 mg

- ✓ Tomato juice - 237 ml - 1.0 mg

Moving on, vitamin B12 is one of the eight B vitamins and is essential for the right formation of the nerves, DNA, and red blood cells. This vitamin provides athletes with energy, so a deficiency in B12 can cause a number of problems including memory loss, paranoia, tingling in the feet and hand, hallucinations, anemia, and fatigue. Vitamin B12 is found rich in animal products including poultry, fish, meat, eggs, and dairy and humans are not able to produce his vitamin on their own.

Plants are not able to produce their own vitamin B12, so vegans and particularly vegan athletes should take extra caution and consume fortified plant foods with B12. In other words, this nutrient is added during the processing of the food. Recommendations are made concerning the B12 vitamin by The Academy of Nutrition and Dietetics for vegetarians and vegans including:

- ✓ "All vegetarians and vegans should be screened for a Vitamin B12 deficiency, through a simple blood test."

- ✓ "All vegans should take a 250 mcg Vitamin B12 supplement daily."

- ✓ "Vegetarians should consider taking 250 mcg B12 supplements a few times per week."

There are various plant foods that are fortified with this vitamin some of them include:

- ✓ Nutritional Yeast - ¼ cup - 17 micrograms of B12

- ✓ Fortified Plant Milks - 1 cup - 3 micrograms of B12 (depending on the brand and variety)

- ✓ Fortified Breakfast Cereal - the amount of vitamin B12 will vary between brands

- ✓ Meat Substitutes - the amount of vitamin B12 will vary depending on the ingredient's list

✓ Nori - the amount of vitamin B12 will vary depending on the ingredient's list and brand.

Various vegan sources of this vitamin are sadly destroyed by cleanliness standards and sterilization processes during the production of foods. For this reason, vegans must check regularly their level of vitamin B12, consume fortified foods with B12, and when necessary, take supplements.

Zinc is essential for our health since it is required for the body to develop over 300 enzymes. This nutrient is the second most richly supplied metal in our bodies after iron. Zinc helps us in enhancing the function of our immune system, in lessening the effects of the common cold, and help in the faster healing of our wounds. A deficiency in zinc can lead to impotence, hinder the time for wound healing, mental fatigue, hair loss, diarrhea, and irregular taste. Vegans should also be cautious of their zinc levels since it is found in a lessened amount in plant foods than in meat and this can also depend on how rich in zinc the soil where the plants grew was. Let us see in more detail vegan foods that are rich in zinc:

✓ Fortified Cereals - 100g - 64 mg

✓ Toasted Wheat Germ - 100g   - 17 mg

✓ Firm Tofu - 100g - 2 mg

✓ Hemp Seeds - 100g - 10 mg

✓ Lentils - 100g - 1 mg

✓ Oatmeal - 100g - 1mg

- ✓ Wild Rice - 100g - 1mg

- ✓ Seeds (Pumpkin and Squash Seeds) - 100g - 8 mg

- ✓ Quinoa - 100g - 1mg

- ✓ Shiitake Mushrooms - 100g - 1 mg

- ✓ Black Beans (Frijoles Negros) - 100g - 1mg

- ✓ Green Peas - 100g - 1 mg

- ✓ Spinach - 100g - 1mg

- ✓ White Button Mushrooms - 100g - 1mg

- ✓ Lima Beans - 100g - 1 mg

- ✓ Chia Seeds - 100g - 5 mg

- ✓ Pecans - 100g - 5 mg

- ✓ Avocados - 100g - 1 mg

- ✓ Flax Seeds - 100g - 4 mg

- ✓ Asparagus - 100g - 1 mg

There are various ways of introducing enough calcium to your vegan and achieving the necessary daily intake for you by following a balanced diet that is filled with foods dense in nutrients, by adding foods fortified with calcium, or if recommended taking supplements. There are various commercial foods like cereals, soy milks, juices, bread products, and tofu that are supplemented with calcium, but to be sure of that, you should read the nutrition labels. Keep in mind that the recommended intake of calcium on a daily bases for women and men between the ages of 19 to 50 years old is 1000 mg.

Calcium plays an essential role in our bodies since it is a fact that it is able to build and preserve our bone. There are several plant foods that contain calcium, so most vegans should be able to meet the daily recommendations. Also, just to be on the safe side, you should check out occasionally your calcium levels, in case you will need supplementation. Let us see the top vegan foods that are rich in calcium:

Soy Foods:

Naturally, soybeans are rich in calcium. For instance, 175 grams or else one cup of soybeans that are cooked will provide you with 1.5% of the recommended daily intake. The same amount of immature soybeans that are otherwise known as edamame will provide you with approximately 27.6% of your recommended daily intake.

Also, the foods that have been made with soybeans like natto, tofu, and tempeh, are rich in calcium too. Tofu that is created with calcium phosphate will have 350 mg per 100 grams. Natto and tempeh that are produced from fermented soybeans will offer us a considerable amount of calcium too. For example, 100 grams of tempeh will be enough to fill 11% of the recommended daily intake while natto will provide you with double that amount.

Lentils, Beans, Peas:

Lentils and beans are also good sources for obtaining calcium, except for fiber and protein. There are different varieties for you to consider that are able o provide you with high levels of calcium per 175 grams. Let us see which will give you the highest:

Winged beans: fill 26% of the Recommended Daily Intake

- ✓ White beans: fill 13% of the Recommended Daily Intake

- ✓ Navy beans: fill 13% of the Recommended Daily Intake

- ✓ Black beans: fill 11% of the Recommended Daily Intake

- ✓ Chickpeas: fill 9% of the Recommended Daily Intake

- ✓ Kidney beans: fill 7% of the Recommended Daily Intake

- ✓ Lentils: fill 4% of the Recommended Daily Intake

An added benefit for you could be that lentils and beans are rich in other nutrients too such as potassium, zinc, folate, iron, and magnesium. However, keep in mind that they also have antinutrients such as lectins and phytates which will lessen the ability of your body to absorb all the other nutrients. According to the study, "Changes in levels of phytic acid, lectins and oxalates during soaking and cooking of Canadian pulses," by Shi L, Arntfield SD, Nickerson M.

You will be able to reduce the levels of those antinutrients by fermenting, soaking, and sprouting lentils and beans. One last thing to keep in mind is that diets which are rich in peas, lentils, and beans, will lower LDL which is bad cholesterol and lessen your risk of developing conditions such as type 2 diabetes, premature death, and heart disease.

Certain Nuts:

It is a fact that all nuts have calcium in small amounts, however, almonds are particularly rich in this mineral since it provides us with 97 mg per 35 grams or else approximately 10% of the recommended daily intake. The second place of nuts rich in calcium goes to Brazil nuts that provide us with about 6% of the recommended daily intake per 35 grams.

Nuts can also offer us healthy fats, proteins, and fiber. They have considerable amounts of B vitamins, selenium, vitamin E and K, copper, magnesium, potassium, and they are rich in antioxidants. By regularly eating nuts, they will offer you the following benefits for your health: help you lower your blood pressure, lessen the risks o developing type 2 diabetes and heart disease, as well as help you lose weight.

 Seeds:

Seeds, as well as their butter, are able to provide us with calcium, but the amount of this mineral they contain will depend on the variety. For example, tahini, which is butter created by sesame seeds, has the most amount of calcium in this category with 130 mg per 30 ml, or else 13% of the recommended daily intake. On the other hand, the same amount of sesame seeds, 20 grams, will only offer us 2% of the recommended daily intake. Flax and chia seeds also include considerable amounts of calcium and provide us with approximately 5 to 6% of the recommended daily intake per 20 to 25 grams.

As is the case with nuts, seeds will also offer us minerals, proteins, fiber, healthy fats, minerals, beneficial plant compounds, and vitamins. They are also connected to health benefits like reduced blood sugar levels, risks of developing heart disease, and reduced inflammation.

Certain Grains:

Generally, grain isn't thought to be a source of calcium, however, some varieties of grain have significant amounts of calcium. For instance, teff and amaranth, which are both ancient grain and free of gluten, will provide you with about 12% of the recommended daily intake per 250 grams or else per each cooked cup. They are both also rich in fiber and can be included in many different dishes. For example, teff can be added to chili after turning it into porridge and amaranth will be an adequate substitute for couscous and rice. You can ground them both into flour and use them to thicken sauces and soups.

Seaweed:

By adding seaweed to your diet, you will be able to increase your intake of calcium. For instance, wakame, which is a seaweed variety that is most commonly consumed when raw, it will offer you approximately 126 mg of calcium or else 12% of your recommended daily intake per each cup or 80 grams. You will be able to find it in almost every Asian supermarket or, for certain, in a sushi restaurant.

Another variety of seaweed that is named kelp can be consumed dried or raw, and it can be another source of calcium since 80 grams of it, or one cup, will provide you with 14% of your recommended daily intake and can be added to main dishes as well as salads. Seaweed can also be a great source of heavy metals. For example, kelp has great amounts of iodine per each portion of about 80 grams, or else one cup.

As you are able to see, there are many sources of nutrients in a vegan diet and when you have a plan and a balanced diet in your hand, you will be able to gain all the health benefits this diet has for your mind, body, and the environment. As for the concern of many athletes about being able to have all the necessary nutrients for them when following a vegan diet, they should be put to rest because a balanced vegan diet will be able to provide you with the appropriate intake of nutrients with only one exception that can be vitamin B12. For this you may need supplements, but keep in mind that there are also people following omnivorous diets that also need supplements of this vitamin.

Vegan Athletes: Meal Plan, Recipes and Advice

When it comes to athletes there are some basic rules that still apply even after you choose to make a transition to the vegan diet. An athlete's body is like a machine that has to deal with the stress of hard and long workouts, everyday stress, as well as stress caused by sleep deprivation due to the long workouts before a big game. For these reasons, nutrition is essential to achieve higher performance and provide it with ways to deal with the stress caused by the different factors we mentioned. The necessary nutrients will not change even if you alter the way you eat and whether you follow an omnivorous or vegan diet you must make sure your sports, nutrition, as well as your habits, are helping you achieve your dreams.

The first thing you should keep in mind is that you should not work out when your stomach is empty. If you were not able to eat within two hours before your training, you could grab a fruit such as one banana or something else that is recommended by your sports dietitian in order for you to keep your blood sugar on a steady level. If your workout is short, for instance it lasts 45 minutes, generally, a piece of fruit will be enough.

You will just have to make sure that your stomach is familiar with this fruit so as to digest it easily. When you have longer workouts, that last for 60 to 90 minutes, you will need to be hydrated appropriately and add more carbs so as to ensure their constant flow. If your workout lasts for over 90 or 120 minutes, you will need a combination of solid food and liquid hydration. For instance, you could eat a bar, boiled potato, or rice.

A rule that applies to everyone, and especially athletes, is that you should not skip your breakfast. This rule exists for a reason. Breakfast will set the pace for your body to use nutrients throughout the rest of the whole day. It is an often occurrence to hear people say that they are not hungry when they wake up and prepare for the day. This is perfectly acceptable, but you shouldn't be on an empty stomach since fueling your body is essential to have energy. Even little things could be added to your breakfast, so as to start building an appetite that could later turn into a full and fitting breakfast. For example, you could have a fruit or prepare a smoothie. You should start small and be consistent on your breakfast for about a week to let your body get used to obtaining nutrients during the morning. From then on you will be able to indulge in a delicious breakfast that will fuel your body with energy.

You should plan out all the meals of 2 to 3 days before your game, so as to ensure that your body will have all the necessary nutrients it needs for your big event by topping its energy and to be certain that you will be at your optimal performance. We see many athletes overlooking this fact and later they feel dizzy or lethargic on such an important day.

To make this planning step easier, you could consult with your sports dietician and include foods that you like and will not cause any distress to your stomach. Keep in mind, that you should not include foods that are high in fiber and saturated fat. You could make a combination of carbs and proteins with a carb to protein ratio of 2:1 or else 3:1 to ensure that your blood sugar levels and proteins stay in check. Another way that you could enforce this is by cooking your meals ahead of time.

Another thing you should keep in mind is that you should never skip your recovery nutrition, in other words meal. If you do this, you will fail in producing results that you strove so hard to achieve throughout your training program. By either consulting with a sports dietician or by yourself, you should figure out which recovery process works best for your training and make it happen within 30 to 45 minutes after your training is over.

You should also eat 90 minutes after that meal and your performance will be at its peak. But why you should eat after 30 to 45 minutes after training? According to experts, that recovery time will expire after 45 to 60 minutes and you will feel more tired and depleted of energy if you skip this. Recovery nutrition in its liquid form appears to be easier for the stomach and it is digested more easily. It also comes in handy when you are not at home to prepare any solid food. You could prepare a drink that is full of proteins or with some amino acids to consume after your training. When you return home, you could prepare a meal with equally distributed amounts of proteins, omega fats, complex carbs, and vegetables. This will stabilize again your blood sugar and keep your body energized.

Last but not least, before you go to sleep, you should consume a snack dense with nutrients and that includes some berries, healthy fats, nuts, and proteins. Generally, foods that will not elevate your blood sugar levels but at the same time protect it from dropping throughout the night. There is a belief that you should not eat before going to bed and it mostly satisfies phycological needs that have to do with self-control and believing that we are not overeating.

However, when it comes to sports nutrition there is little psychological benefit from fasting before going to sleep. It is a fact the level of blood sugar will fall rapidly during sleep to maintain the processes of the body. If we do not fuel it with nutrients, the body will have nothing to rebuild from. You shouldn't ask yourself if you should eat or not, but rather what type of food would be best for you during a particular time of the day. The body of athletes is moving constantly and thus it will constantly need refueling to rebuilt itself. One of the worst things athletes of any kind could do is to restrict their intake f nutrients and hope to get an improved performance through that.

You shouldn't be stressed when it comes to eating right in order to attain the nutrients you need. For instance, you can build a framework with seven foods that feel most important to you or your sports dietician and try to include them in your diet for each day throughout the week. An example of such a framework can be:

Cruciferous Vegetables and Leafy Greens: An amazing addition to your vegan diet that is very beneficial for your health.

Berries and Other Fruit: They present us with the most vibrant colors and have anti-inflammatory, anti-cancer, and antioxidant properties.

Flaxseeds and Other Seeds and Nuts: Walnuts and flaxseeds are rich in Omega-3 and also flaxseeds are antiangiogenic.

Beans: According to a 2007 American Institute for Cancer Research study we should consume beans every day for their many health benefits.

White or Green Tea: Tea is rich in antioxidants and also includes beneficial phytochemicals such as ECGC that are exclusive to the tea bush.

Garlic and Onions: According to research half a cup of onions each day is able to reduce the risk of certain cancers by 50-80%. Garlic would be an added plus.

Tumeric: It is able to help us against cancer and heart disease due to its curcumin and pigment.

The above is an example of a framework for you to work with and add foods that benefit you and you would love to eat each day. However, it can be difficult for most people to think of ways to incorporate those foods into their meals. Admittedly it is a hard part, especially for extremely busy athletes. To solve this problem, you could at first try to add those foods into your three basic meals. As an example, we will take the foods mentioned above and try to include them into the three basic meals, breakfast, lunch, and dinner:

Breakfast:

You can make a morning smoothie or oatmeal that will include some of the foods of your framework before you start your day. For example, you can have:

Other Fruit and Berries

Other nuts and Flaxseeds

White or green Tea Leaves

Beans

Tumeric

Lunch:

For lunch, you can have a big bowl of salad with a number of vegetables, beans, greens, and create a dressing based with nuts such as tahini with garlic or cashew ranch. In this salad you can include:

Seeds and Nuts

Onions

Greens

Beans

Cruciferous Vegetables

Fruit

Tumeric

Whole Grain

Dinner:

You will have many choices for dinner when you base it around greens, grain, and beans. For example, you can have tacos and burritos, curries, pasta, and combine them with garlic or onions. The foods you could include in dinner are:

Greens

Mushrooms

Cruciferous or other Vegetables

Turmeric

Beans

Whole Grain

Seeds and nuts as dressing or topping

Garlic and Onion

When we place all the foods together we can create a sample meal plan for a day which will include all the foods of your framework along with other foods such as mushrooms, and whole grains. Keep in mind that your ideal meal plan would be better if you included the seven foods of your choice at the proportions your sports dietician should indicate. A sample meal plan includes:

Breakfast: A smoothie with additionally tea, water, or coffee

Morning Snack: Tea, fruit with an optional addition of nut butter.

133

Lunch: A big salad with beans and a dressing based on nuts. Optionally you could use at the side whole grain such as whole-wheat bread, quinoa, or rice.

Afternoon Snack: Whole grain, such as bread or crackers, or veggies with hummus and tea.

Dinner: Foods that contain beans, grain, and green with garlic and onion.

If required, you may need supplements of vitamin D3, B12, and DHA/EPA. Diets that are based on plants and whole-food, even though they are high in various micronutrients, they do not offer enough vitamin D3, B12, and DHA/EPA. You can get these three nutrients from a single source if it is recommended and also keep in mind that there are people who follow omnivorous diets that lack those vitamins too. It is just that vegans may be at a higher risk of developing a deficiency in them due to the complete lack of animal food. Let us see in more detail a few recipes that will help you in preparing your three basic meals.

Recipes for Breakfast:

Banana and Berry Smoothie:

Smoothies are an easy way, through which you will be able to obtain the nutrients you need for breakfast. You can make smoothies with blueberries, strawberries, and blackberries or any other fruit you like. It could also help you experimenting with different fruit so as to not get bored with the taste.

Ingredients:

- ✓ 2 medium-sized and ripe bananas
- ✓ 2 spoonful of walnuts or Brazil nuts
- ✓ 2 spoonful of flaxseeds
- ✓ 2 ½ cups of water
- ✓ 2 ½ cups of frozen berry
- ✓ 2 baby spinach or any other greens soft in taste

Optional:

- ✓ Green tea leaves
- ✓ Fresh turmeric
- ✓ Tofu

Instructions:

Pour all the ingredients in a blender and blend until they get smooth.

Oatmeal:

- ✓ 1 cup of oats
- ✓ ¼ spoonful of cinnamon
- ✓ 2 cups of water
- ✓ 1 spoonful of grounded flaxseeds

- ✓ ½ cup of frozen berries

- ✓ 1 spoonful of chia seeds

- ✓ ¼ cup of grounded almonds

- ✓ 3 spoonful of pumpkin seeds

- ✓ Maple syrup for taste - optional

Instructions:

- ✓ Place the oats, cinnamon, and water together in a saucepan that is in medium heat.

- ✓ Heat the ingredients until they are simmering, and stir often until the water is absorbed which takes approximately five minutes.

- ✓ Pour in and stir the flaxseeds and berries until they are heated enough and then, take them off the heat.

- ✓ Pour the end result in a bowl and top it with pumpkin seeds, maple syrup, chia seeds, and almonds.

<u>Recipes for Lunch</u>:

For lunch you can create a rich salad with various dressings that is full of cruciferous veggies, greens, grain, seeds, and beans. The dressing you can top it with could be free of oil and based on nuts for added taste. Let us see in more detail how to create an amazing salad:

Instructions:

Cut one large lettuce and add a handful of the following:

- ✓ Arugula

- ✓ Dandelion greens

- ✓ Baby kale

- ✓ Mustard Greens

Add at least one of the cruciferous vegetables such as:

- ✓ Cabbage

- ✓ Radishes

- ✓ Broccoli

Add also green onions as well as any other of the vegetables you like such as

- ✓ Tomatoes

- ✓ Carrots

- ✓ Celery

Finish the salad with a cup of beans as well as a dressing that is based on nuts. You will be able to serve this salad with brown rice or with whole-grain sides to fill you more. Let us see how you will be able to make two dressings that are delicious with a salad.

137

<u>Tahini and Garlic Dressing</u>:

Ingredients:

- ✓ ½ cup of tahini

- ✓ 2 cloves of garlic or more for your taste

- ✓ ¼ cup of water and if needed more for thinner results

- ✓ 2 spoonfuls of lemon juice

- ✓ 2 spoonfuls of tamari reduced in sodium

Instructions:

- ✓ Toss the garlic cloves after you peel them over medium heat in a dry skillet for 5 to 10 minutes up until they have taken a light brown color. This will help take down the intensity of the garlic a bit and retain its flavor.

- ✓ Add the garlic to your food processor blender and mince them.

- ✓ Then, add the other ingredients to the blender and mince them until they are smooth. Add the water until you achieve a thin texture, but not so thin that it will not stick to the salad leaves.

- ✓ Keep in mind that it will thicken in the fridge too, so you could always add more water before you actually use it.

- ✓ If you feel that the flavor is too strong, you could add extra Tahini or water.

<u>Cashew Ranch Dressing</u>:

Ingredients:

- ✓ 1 and ¼ cups of cashews - you can soak them if you want a creamier dressing

- ✓ 1 cup of water to blend

- ✓ 1 and 1/2 spoonful of lemon juice

- ✓ 1 spoonful of apple cider vinegar

- ✓ ½ spoonful of garlic powder

- ✓ 1.5 spoonful of onion powder

- ✓ 1 spoonful of dried dill

- ✓ 1 spoonful of sea salt

- ✓ ½ spoonful of dried basil

- ✓ ¼ spoonful of freshly grounded black pepper

Instructions:

- ✓ You should blend all the ingredients in a high-speed blender up until they are smooth and creamy to suit your taste.

- ✓ Keep in mind that you should not blend them for too long since the dressing will get hot. If it is too thick for your taste, you could add more water.

✓ Another thing to keep in mind is that it will thicken more in the fridge; if this happens, add more water to it.

<u>Recipes for Dinner</u>:

An appropriate dinner could be rice, pasta, tacos or stews, and many more foods of your choice that include:

✓ Garlic and Onions

✓ Whole Grain

✓ Beans

✓ Greens

✓ Seeds and Nuts

✓ Turmeric

✓ Vegetables

✓ Mushrooms

Let us see in more detail an amazing recipe that will make you full and that tastes great:

<u>Tempeh Tacos</u>:

Keep in mind that if you don't like soy, you will be able to replace it with any other bean.

Ingredients:

140

- ✓ 454 grams of crumbled tempeh

- ✓ 12 corn tortillas

- ✓ Soy sauce or tamari low in sodium

- ✓ 340 grams of BBQ sauce - preferably without oil

- ✓ 1 cup of shredded green or red cabbage

- ✓ ½ bunch of chopped and fresh cilantro

- ✓ 1 cup of chopped pineapple

- ✓ pickled onions for garnish

- ✓ Serrano pepper or Jalapeño

Instructions:

- ✓ Use a medium pan and preheat it over medium to high heat.

- ✓ Once it is warm enough, heat each corn tortilla for one minute on one side and then flip it to heat the other side for approximately 10 seconds.

- ✓ After you heat each tortilla, place it on a plate that is covered by an almost damp kitchen towel in order to maintain its warmth.

- ✓ Use a pan to heat over medium heat the crumbled tempeh and stir it often to prevent it from sticking.

✓ Once it is heated, sprinkle the tempeh with soy sauce or tamari sauce and stir it often up until the tempeh is heated thoroughly.

✓ Then, add the barbecue sauce and mix them well until they are heated thoroughly.

✓ To complete this recipe, take a spoonful of the tempeh blend and place it onto a warm tortilla.

✓ Then add the pineapple, red cabbage, jalapeño, pickled onions, and cilantro. Repeat this process for the rest of the tortillas

The above are only a few recipes out of the many others you can find in order to have the best and extremely tasty food on your plate. Many people think that vegan recipes lack many things that would make food delicious and the fact of the matter is that they are completely wrong. Vegan food lacks nothing when compared to food that contains meat and meat by-products. Athletes will be able to taste amazing foods while at the same time maintain all the nutrients they need to be at their peak performance. Vegan foods do not restrict your creativity, on the contrary, they will allow you to unleash your imagination and make foods that will be mouth-dropping, healthy, and environmentally friendly.

Epilogue

As we were able to see throughout the course of this book, the vegan diet is completely healthy and appropriate for athletes and the overall world population. It has many health benefits and includes all the necessary ingredients for us to achieve our optimal health while eating a variety of vegetables, pulses, fruit, seeds as well as fortified foods. There are several myths surrounding the vegan diet including the one that only vegetarians need supplements.

While this may be true to some extent for vitamin B12, even though people who follow omnivorous diets may need supplements too, vegans and people who are not vegan may need supplements like VEG1 to make sure that they are receiving everything they need. For instance, fortified foods are for both vegans and non-vegans to maintain a healthy way of life, so they are not a necessity only for people who follow the vegan diet.

There is also the misconception that being vegan and eating a diet based on plants is the same thing. While it is true that vegans follow a diet based primarily on plants, veganism is much more than just food. People may follow a plant-based diet for health reasons; however, people indulge in veganism mainly because they wish to do no harm to every living being including animals. Vegans do not only exclude animal products from their diets, but they also do not purchase products that are tested on animals, they try to reduce their carbon emissions by recycling, they opt to shop local among many other things. They want the best for the environment and the world in general.

Veganism may seem more challenging to athletes due to concerns about nutrients. There is no need to worry since every athlete is going to get all the nutrients they need through careful planning and consulting a sports dietician regularly. A big mistake most people do when they make the transition to veganism is being too strict with their diet. Our bodies need quality food that provides us with energy, nutrients, as well as calories. No person will be able to function while following restrictive diets no matter if they include meat or not. Vegan diets should not have to include cucumber juice for breakfast or just a raw smoothie for dinner. Keep your vegan diet rich by educating yourself on the many different ways you can work with your food.

Being a vegan will be an amazing choice that will open your mind and promote your health. Be clear on the reason why you want to be a vegan because many people have failed because they simply adopted veganism on a wimp. If, at first, you miss meat, do not give up, it is completely normal. Do not give up on making a significant impact due to a few setbacks. We are not perfect and we will achieve everything we need through hard work and this means learning from our mistakes. Embrace the importance of living a lifestyle free of animal products and cruelty as well as attaining the healthiest version of you.

Bibliography

1. Brenda Davis and Vesanto Melina: Becoming Vegan: The Complete Guide to Adopting a Healthy Plant-Based Diet, April 10, 2000.

2. Victoria Moran and Adair Moran: Main Street Vegan: Everything You Need to Know to Eat Healthfully and Live Compassionately in the Real World, April 26, 2012.

3. Matt Frazier and Matthew Ruscigno: No Meat Athlete: Run on Plants and Discover Your Fittest, Fastest, Happiest Self, October 1, 2013.

4. Erik Marcus: Vegan: The New Ethics of Eating, October 1, 2000.

5. Brendan Brazier: Thrive: The Vegan Nutrition Guide to Optimal Performance in Sports and Life, December 23, 2008.

6. Celine Steen: The Complete Guide to Vegan Food Substitutions: Veganize It! Foolproof Methods for Transforming Any Dish into a Delicious New Vegan Favorite, December 1, 2010.

7. Matt Frazier, Stepfanie Romine, and Rich Roll: The No Meat Athlete Cookbook: Whole Food, Plant-Based Recipes to Fuel Your Workouts—and the Rest of Your Life, May 16, 2017.

8. Ben Greene, Brett Stewart: The Vegan Athlete: Maximizing Your Health and Fitness While Maintaining a Compassionate Lifestyle, January 29, 2013.

9. Nicolas Benfatto: The Vegan Cookbook For Athletes: 45 high-protein delicious recipes for a plant-based diet plan and healthy muscle in bodybuilding, fitness and sports, June 13, 2019.

10. Robert Cheeke and Vanessa Espinoza: Plant-Based Muscle: Our Roadmap to Peak Performance on a Plant-Based Diet, September 2, 2017.